Dynamic Ophthalmic Ultrasonography

A Video Atlas for Ophthalmologists and Imaging Technicians

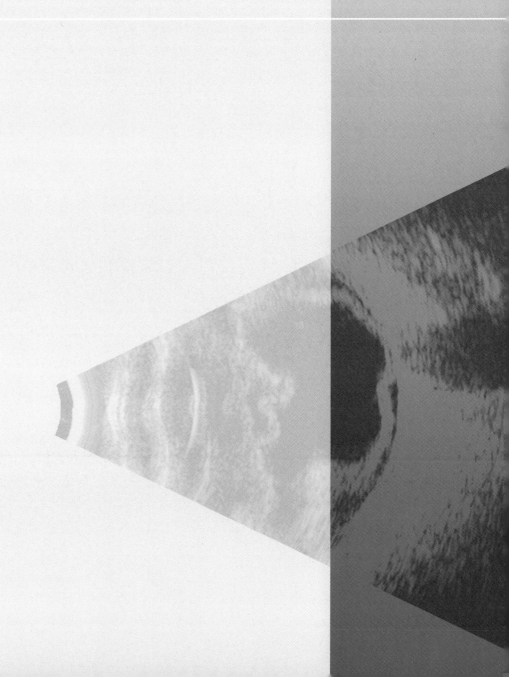

Dynamic Ophthalmic Ultrasonography

A Video Atlas for Ophthalmologists and Imaging Technicians

The Advanced Retinal Imaging Center Collection of The New York Eye & Ear Infirmary

AUTHOR

Julian Pancho S. Garcia Jr., MD

Associate Professor of Ophthalmology
The New York Eye & Ear Infirmary, New York, New York
New York Medical College, Valhalla, New York

ADVISERS

Paul T. Finger, MD, FACS

Associate Professor of Ophthalmology
The New York Eye & Ear Infirmary
New York University School of Medicine
New York, New York

Richard B. Rosen, MD, FACS, FASRS, CRA

Vice-Chairman and Associate Professor of Ophthalmology
The New York Eye & Ear Infirmary, New York, New York
New York Medical College, Valhalla, New York

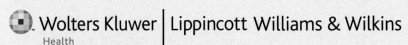

Wolters Kluwer | Lippincott Williams & Wilkins
Health

Philadelphia · Baltimore · New York · London
Buenos Aires · Hong Kong · Sydney · Tokyo

Senior Executive Editor: Jonathan Pine
Marketing Manager: Lisa Lawrence
Senior Product Manager: Emilie Moyer
Senior Designer: Stephen Druding
Production Service: Maryland Composition Inc.

351 West Camden Street
Baltimore, MD 21201

530 Walnut Street
Philadelphia, PA 19106

Printed in China

Library of Congress Cataloging-in-Publication Data

Garcia, Julian Pancho S.
 Dynamic ophthalmic ultrasonography : a video atlas for ophthalmologists and imaging technicians/ Julian Pancho S. Garcia Jr.
  p. ; cm.
 Includes bibliographical references and index.
 ISBN 978-1-60831-143-9
 1. Eye—Ultrasonic imaging—Atlases. I. Title.
 [DNLM: 1. Eye Diseases—ultrasonography—Atlases. 2. Eye—ultrasonography—Atlases. 3. Eye Movements—Atlases. 4. Video Recording—methods—Atlases. WW 17 G216d 2009]
 RE79.U4G37 2009
 617.7'1543—dc22
                                2009014884

To purchase additional copies of this book, call our customer service department at **(800) 638-3030** or fax orders to **(301) 223-2320.** International customers should call **(301) 223-2300.**

Visit Lippincott Williams & Wilkins on the Internet: http://www.LWW.com. Lippincott Williams & Wilkins customer service representatives are available from 8:30 am to 6:00 pm, EST.

06 07 08 09 10
1 2 3 4 5 6 7 8 9 10

To my dearest wife
Patricia

My beloved sons
Santino and Lorenzo

My dear parents
Julian and Nominada

And the rest of my family

Contents

Section III | Case Presentations

Foreword

I n the last 40 years, the advancements in ocular imaging have been most dramatic. From the use of ultrasound when I was a medical resident to determine a midline brain shift, to the spectacular B-scans laboriously produced by Professor Gilbert Baum when I was a Retina Fellow in 1973, new imaging devices such as the ultrasound biomicroscopy (UBM), anterior and posterior slit lamp ophthalmoscopy (SLO), optical coherence tomography (OCT), OCT-SLO, Heidelberg retinal tomography (HRT), and the like, have redrawn the face of ophthalmology. A parallel has been the radiologic evolution from x-rays to computed axial tomography (CAT) and magnetic resonance imaging (MRI).

At The New York Eye & Ear Infirmary, we have been most fortunate in participating in the early phases of anterior segment imaging under the leadership of Professor Robert Ritch, MD, Director of Glaucoma, and posterior segment imaging under the leadership of Professor Richard B. Rosen, MD, Vice-Chairman of Ophthalmology. In addition, the participation of Professor Paul T. Finger, Director of Ocular Oncology, has been most significant.

In this Video Atlas, Dr. Julian Pancho S. Garcia Jr., presents anterior and posterior segment B-scan ultrasonography in a dynamic fashion. Using material gathered over the last 8 years at the Advanced Retinal Imaging Center of The New York Eye & Ear Infirmary, and culling from his vast experience from thousands of clinical cases, he presents the material in a form not only for ophthalmologists, but also for ophthalmic technicians. Dr. Garcia has been able to confirm his interpretation of these cases from clinical information as well as operative outcomes and, occasionally, pathological reports. Thus, he has been able to refine the art of dynamic B-scan ultrasonography and fine-tune his ultrasound acuity in ophthalmology.

He begins each section of this Atlas by teaching the proper techniques to obtain dynamic images, and then goes on to demonstrate the various aspects of normal anatomy and pathology. The various forms of movement of eye tissues as recorded by B-scan ultrasound are illustrated to give the viewer a working knowledge of ophthalmic tissue dynamics and the implications therein.

By utilizing a large selection of videos, Dr. Garcia shows how the understanding of these tissue dynamics can allow the correct diagnostic interpretation of many ocular conditions, with special emphasis on the vitreo-retinal-optic nerve interactions. The single captured photo of a B-scan is shown to be very inadequate in light of these high-quality dynamic videos.

The goal of this text is achieved not by allowing a tutorial in ultrasound interpretation, but by providing a standard to keep on hand so one could immediately compare this standard to a clinical case.

I am sure this *Video Atlas of Dynamic Ophthalmic Ultrasonography* will be a valuable addition to all dealing with this subject.

Joseph B. Walsh, MD
Professor and Chairman
Department of Ophthalmology
The New York Eye & Ear Infirmary
New York Medical College
New York, New York

Preface

This video atlas was written to complement the existing literature on ophthalmic ultrasonography. In particular, it is a dynamic presentation of various ophthalmic and orbital entities that may be encountered in a clinical setting, such as The New York Eye & Ear Infirmary (NYEEI). The atlas does not attempt to discuss the clinicopathogenesis of ophthalmic conditions and disease entities that are included in the collection. Rather, it is envisioned to be a video guide, especially for ophthalmologists and imaging technicians wishing to learn more about what has been excellently written and extensively covered in today's reference textbooks. It brings to life what these books have attempted to describe in words.

The book is designed to be a reference tool in a clinical setting. For the very first time in ophthalmic literature, it dynamically presents the basic ultrasound movements observed in the eye and orbit. Each ophthalmic tissue demonstrates a specific type of motion unique and inherent to its anatomic structure. This basic movement may change, however, as a result of inflammatory or degenerative factors, or the presence of other associated findings. Consequently, the motion displayed may no longer be normal for that tissue and may resemble the basic movement of a different anatomic structure, leading to confusion and errors in diagnosis. This is where the importance of the video atlas comes in. It presents the usual movement of a particular tissue, and then shows the possible types of motion it could manifest in various pathologic situations. In other words, the reader is provided with visual information about typical and atypical tissue movements. By repeatedly watching the movies in the collection, one becomes familiar with how ophthalmic tissues behave, and with exposure to the intricacies of ophthalmic tissue dynamics, the reader becomes adept at recognizing which specific anatomic structures are involved when confronted with a similar case the next time around. Eventually, he or she learns to interpret ultrasound findings in a more logical manner and, hopefully, one can more proficiently arrive at sound ultrasound interpretation. This is the practical objective of the video atlas. Toward the end of the book, a number of cases are presented to gauge what has been learned from the previous sections.

At this point, allow me to thank my wife, Patricia, for her much-needed support and invaluable insight, as well as my sons, Santino and Lorenzo, for their patience and understanding when I wrote the book and put the atlas together. Likewise, I am deeply grateful to Katy W. Tai, Clinical Research Manager of The NYEEI, and Catherine M. Pannone, Assistant Nursing Care Coordinator of the Retina Center, for their sound advice and encouragement.

Julian Pancho S. Garcia Jr., MD

SECTION I

Overview

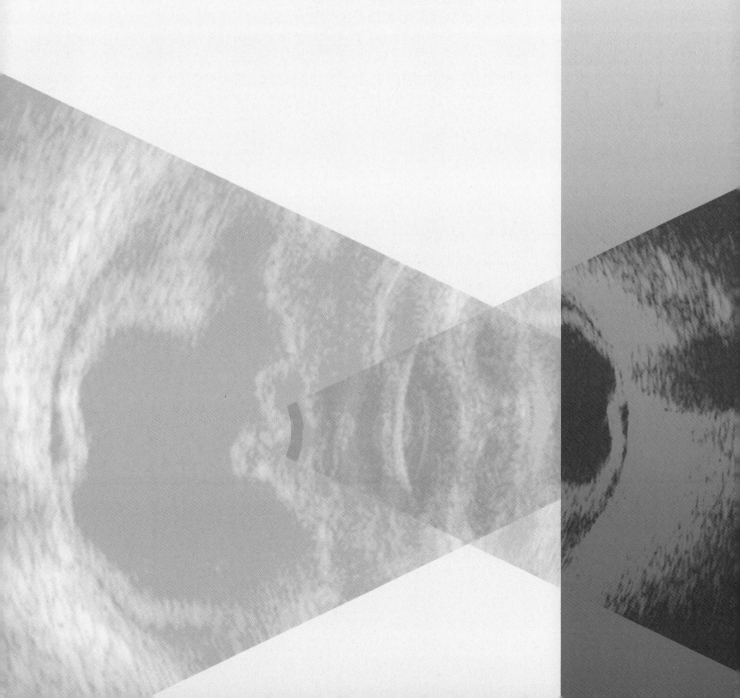

Introduction

"A picture is worth a thousand words." A movie, on the other hand, is worth a thousand pictures. Words cannot accurately depict motion as well as a movie can, no matter how descriptive the choice of words. Nowhere is this statement more appropriate than in the black-and-white setting of ophthalmic ultrasonography, where still images cannot adequately convey the true picture without revealing the element of motion present within each and every ophthalmic condition.

For more than three decades now, B-scan ultrasonography has played a key role as a valuable diagnostic imaging device in the field of Ophthalmology.[1] Beginning with the more invasive fluid-immersion technique of the past, B-scan has now evolved to be less intrusive, utilizing the contact method of the present system. B-scan ultrasound makes use of a transducer that emits ultrasound waves ranging from 10–20 MHz for posterior segment imaging to 35–50 MHz for anterior segment imaging, scanning the eye to produce a two-dimensional (2D), cross-sectional image. The ultrasound picture that is generated is commonly referred to as the 2D B-scan for posterior segment imaging, or ultrasound biomicroscope (UBM) scan for anterior segment imaging.

Ophthalmic ultrasound movements have been classified into three basic forms: convection, aftermovement, and vascularity.[1] These types of echographic motion are traditionally depicted as a succession of fuzzy ultrasound spikes on an A-scan image, or as a change in the position of tissues on a sequence of 2D B-scan images. However, neither the captured image of A- or B-scan ultrasound can adequately represent the ultrasound movements that are actually seen and observed during the acquisition of these images. Similarly, three-dimensional (3D) ophthalmic ultrasound imaging assembles a series of still 2D B-scans to form a 3D image block for interactive analysis. However, there exists no dynamic component to the acquired 3D images, unless and until ophthalmic "real time" 3D imaging becomes available.[2] Recently, real time digital 2D B-scan video recording has become the preferred mode of capturing ultrasound images in many 2D and 3D ultrasound systems, and this has provided the ophthalmic community a valuable means to demonstrate as well as document the ophthalmic tissue dynamics of many interesting cases in the clinics.

This video collection is, therefore, presented as a practical guide for ophthalmologists and imaging technicians on various ultrasound movements that may be observed in the eye and orbit. A working knowledge of ophthalmic tissue dynamics is essential in confidently unraveling the differential diagnosis of ophthalmic conditions and disease entities, necessary for making an accurate ultrasound interpretation of clinical cases.

HOW TO OBTAIN DYNAMIC OPHTHALMIC ULTRASOUND MOVIES

Anterior Ocular Segment

Dynamic ultrasound studies involving the anterior ocular segment are specifically indicated for light-and-dark tests in glaucoma, where video images of the angle are obtained utilizing the fluid-immersion technique of UBM. After numbing the surface of the eye with a topical anesthetic, a rubberized eyecup is inserted between the lids. About ⅔ of the eyecup is filled with contact lens solution, preferably using solutions formulated for sensitive eyes. This cup is held against the globe with just enough pressure to prevent leakage of fluid from the eye. A 35 or 50 MHz high frequency ultrasound probe is used for this purpose, dipped in the fluid and held in position over the angle of interest during ultrasound scanning.

Posterior Ocular Segment and Orbit

Dynamic ultrasound studies involving the posterior ocular segment and orbit are generally indicated for various conditions requiring clinical documentation and/or diagnostic verification. Here, topical anesthetic drops are applied on the ocular surface. The tip of a regular 10, 12, or 12.5 MHz B-scan probe is coated with conductive electrode gel, and is held in position on the surface of the lid or directly on the globe during ultrasound scanning. Note that the use of a high resolution 20 MHz B-scan probe is not recommended for dynamic ultrasound examinations, since it cannot highlight details of the vitreous cavity as effectively as a 10, 12, or 12.5 MHz B-scan probe.

POSITIONING OF THE PROBE

The Probe

The ultrasound probe is a unique imaging instrument. It generates a 2D ultrasound scan from the arc-like oscillation of the transducer tip. The ultrasound probe can be likened to a flashlight used to visualize either the anterior or posterior segments of the eye. It can be pointed in any direction, depending on the part of the eye you wish to examine. Unlike a regular flashlight which shines a conical beam, the ultrasound probe casts a slit beam. Hence, one can only see a linear image of the ophthalmic structure that the beam falls on. The slit ultrasound beam penetrates the eye to provide a view not only of the surface and structures above it, but also structures located beneath it. This slice of structures above and beneath the surface of the eye is what is referred to as a 2D, cross-sectional ultrasound view.

The ultrasound probe for anterior segment imaging (UBM) has an exposed transducer tip, while the transducer for posterior segment imaging (B-scan) is located within the tip of the probe (Fig.1-1). In both probes, a marker is present on the sleeve close to the transducer tip which serves as a guide for imaging orientation purposes.

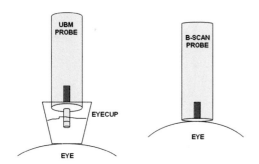

Figure 1-1 A UBM probe has an exposed transducer that is dipped in a cup of eye solution for imaging. A B-scan probe has a transducer within its tip and is placed on the eye or lid for imaging using a conductive gel. Both probes have a marker for imaging orientation purposes.

The marker on the probe corresponds to the top of the scan plane (Fig.1-2). Thus, when the probe is held with the marker positioned superiorly, the transducer oscillates and scans along a vertical direction, cutting across the anterior (UBM) or posterior (B-scan) segment of the eye. In this instance, the top of the oscillation arc is the top of the scan plane.

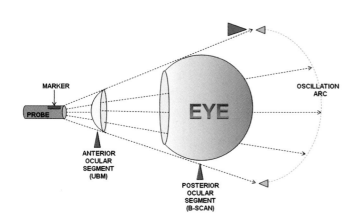

Figure 1-2 When the ultrasound probe is positioned with the marker on top, the transducer oscillates along a vertical arc (dashed orange line) and casts a slit beam across the surface of the anterior or posterior ocular segment. Here, the top of the oscillation arc is the top of the scan plane (blue arrowhead).

The scan plane is likewise vertical even when the marker is positioned inferiorly (Fig.1-3). This time, the bottom of the oscillation arc is the top of the scan plane.

Figure 1-3 When the ultrasound probe is positioned with the marker below, the transducer still oscillates along a vertical arc (dashed orange line) and casts a slit beam across the surface of the anterior or posterior ocular segment. Here, the bottom of the oscillation arc is the top of the scan plane (blue arrowhead).

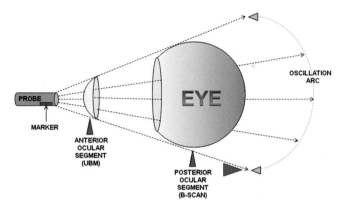

The same thing applies when the marker is positioned towards the left or the right side, and the transducer oscillates horizontally. The top of the oscillation arc corresponds to the right or the left side of the scan plane, respectively.

TIP

The marker on the ultrasound probe always corresponds to the top of the scan plane.

The Ultrasound Scan

The ultrasound scan, which is also termed echogram, is a 2D representation of the eye generated by the oscillation of the ultrasound beam (Fig.1-4). In anterior ocular segment imaging, the marker corresponds to the left side of any UBM scan. In posterior ocular segment imaging, the marker corresponds to the top of any 2D B-scan image. This rule is regardless of where the marker is positioned.

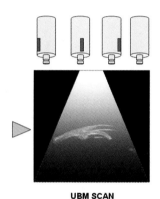

UBM SCAN

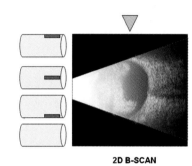

2D B-SCAN

Figure 1-4 Regardless of where the marker is positioned, the marker on the probe always corresponds to the left side of a UBM scan or the top of a 2D B-scan image (orange arrowhead).

TIP

As a rule, the marker on the ultrasound probe corresponds to the left side of any UBM scan or the top of any 2D B-scan image, regardless of where the marker is positioned.

The Eye

The eye can be likened to a face of the clock, where the top is 12 o'clock, the right side is 3 o'clock, the bottom is 6 o'clock, and the left side is 9 o'clock (Fig.1-5). These points of reference are the same whether one is performing anterior or posterior ocular segment imaging, or scanning the right or the left eye. Therefore, the superior angle (anterior ocular segment imaging) or superior fundus (posterior ocular segment imaging) is always 12 o'clock, while the inferior angle (anterior ocular segment imaging) or inferior fundus (posterior ocular segment imaging) is always 6 o'clock in either eye.

Figure 1-5 Vertical Points of Reference

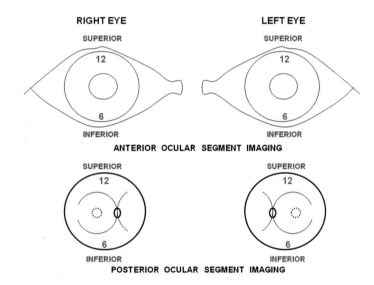

TIP

In anterior and posterior ocular segment imaging, the top is 12 o'clock and the bottom is 6 o'clock in both eyes.

Confusion may arise when viewing the 3 o'clock and 9 o'clock points of reference. Keep in mind that the right eye is a mirror image of the left eye (Fig.1-6). Hence, the nasal angle (anterior ocular segment imaging) or nasal fundus (posterior ocular segment imaging) is 3 o'clock in the right eye and 9 o'clock in the left eye. Conversely, the temporal angle (anterior ocular segment imaging) or temporal fundus (posterior ocular segment imaging) is 9 o'clock in the right eye and 3 o'clock in the left eye.

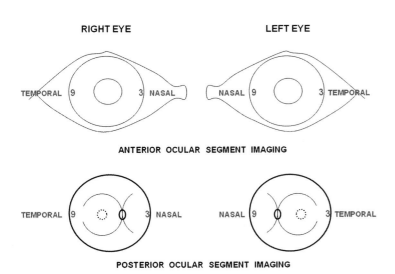

Figure 1-6 Horizontal Points of Reference

> **TIP**
>
> In anterior and posterior ocular segment imaging, the nasal side is 3 o'clock in the right and 9 o'clock in the left eye, while the temporal side is 9 o'clock in the right and 3 o'clock in the left eye. Think mirror image.

ANTERIOR OCULAR SEGMENT IMAGING

There are three ways to image the anterior ocular segment: radial, transverse, and axial views.

In radial views of the angle, the probe is positioned over the limbus with the marker facing away from the center of the cornea. Thus, the left side of the scan is the limbal side, while the right is the central corneal side. There are as many radial views as there are hours in a clock. Radial views are imaged directly over the angle of interest. Figure 1-7 shows how a radial view of the 9 o'clock angle is obtained in the right eye.

Figure 1-7   Radial View of the 9 o'clock Angle (Right Eye)

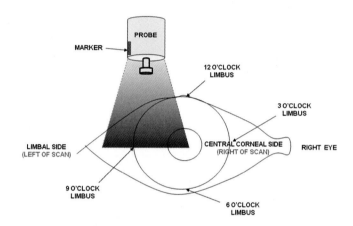

Transverse and axial views of the anterior ocular segment are not used in this atlas and are therefore not discussed here. For further information on anterior ocular segment views, please refer to the book on UBM mentioned at the end of the book.

TIP

In radial views of the angle, the marker is always positioned away from the center of the cornea.

Mnemonic: RADIAL for RADIAL AWAY.

POSTERIOR OCULAR SEGMENT IMAGING

For the posterior ocular segment and orbit, there are three ways to image the eye: axial, transverse, and longitudinal views.

Axial Views

Horizontal axial views allow simultaneous imaging of the lens, optic nerve, and the macula. In this view, the tip of the probe is placed at the center of the cornea, with the marker positioned toward the nasal side of the eye. Thus, the top of the scan is the nasal side, while the bottom is the temporal side. Figure 1-8 illustrates how a horizontal axial view of the right eye is taken. A horizontal axial view of the left eye is simply a mirror image of the right eye, as shown in Figure 1-9.

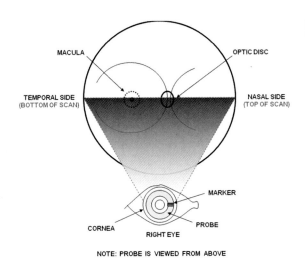

Figure 1-8 Horizontal Axial View (Right Eye)

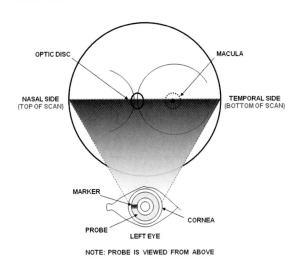

Figure 1-9 Horizontal Axial View (Left Eye)

Vertical axial views provide simultaneous imaging of the lens and the optic nerve. In this view, the tip of the probe is placed at the center of the cornea, with the marker positioned toward the superior side of the eye. Thus, the top of the scan is the superior side, while the bottom is the inferior side, as shown in Figure 1-10, an illustration of the right eye.

Figure 1-10 Vertical Axial View (Right Eye)

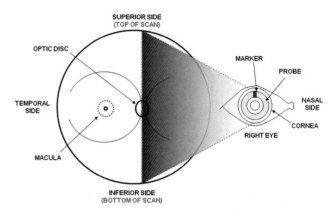

One can twist the probe 45 degrees to the right or 45 degrees to the left to obtain oblique axial views of the eye. Similar to vertical axial views, the marker is always positioned at the superior side. Oblique axial views are not used in this book and are not discussed here. For further discussion about oblique axial views, please refer to the suggested readings included at the end of the book.

Furthermore, one can obtain an axial view of the eye just above or below the level of the optic nerve head, as well as immediately to the right or to the left of it. These are termed para-axial views of the eye. Figure 1-11 depicts how a horizontal para-axial view just above the level of the optic nerve head is recorded in the left eye.

Figure 1-11 Horizontal Para-axial View (Left Eye)

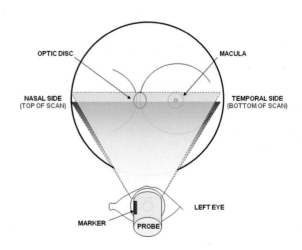

Figure 1-12, on the other hand, shows how a vertical para-axial view immediately to the left of the optic nerve head is taken in the right eye.

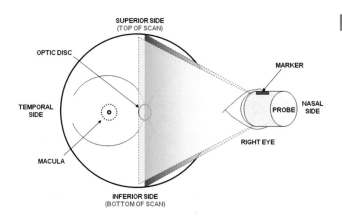

Figure 1-12 Vertical Para-axial View (Right Eye)

Transverse Views

Transverse views provide a lateral sweep of one quadrant of the fundus. Like the radial views (anterior ocular segment imaging), there are as many transverse views as there are hours in a clock.

In horizontal transverse views, the tip of the probe is placed on the sclera below the cornea pointing up to view the superior fundus, or on the sclera above the cornea pointing down to view the inferior fundus. Like the horizontal axial view, the marker is always positioned at the nasal side of the eye. Thus, the top of the scan is the nasal side, while the bottom is the temporal side. Figure 1-13 demonstrates how a horizontal transverse view of the superior fundus is captured in the right eye.

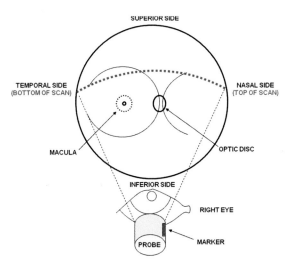

Figure 1-13 Horizontal Transverse View of the Superior Fundus (Right Eye)

In vertical transverse views, the tip of the probe is placed on the sclera nasal to the cornea pointing toward the opposite side of the eye to view the temporal fundus. Alternatively, the probe is placed on the sclera temporal to the cornea pointing toward the opposite side to view the nasal fundus. Like the vertical axial view, the marker is always positioned at the superior side of the eye. Hence, the top of the scan is the superior side, while the bottom is the inferior side. Figure 1-14 shows how a vertical transverse view of the temporal fundus is obtained in the right eye.

Figure 1-14 Vertical Transverse View of the Temporal Fundus (Right Eye)

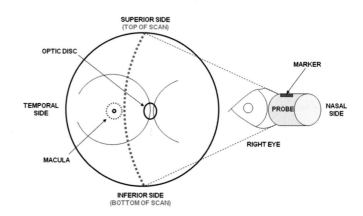

In both horizontal and vertical transverse views, one can point the probe toward the back of the eye (posterior to the equator) to obtain a more posterior transverse view of the fundus. Alternatively, one can point the probe toward the front (anterior to the equator) to obtain a more peripheral transverse view of the fundus. Figure 1-15 demonstrates how a peripheral vertical transverse view of the temporal fundus is recorded in the right eye.

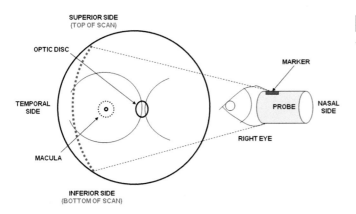

Figure 1-15 Peripheral Vertical Transverse View of the Temporal Fundus (Right Eye)

Oblique transverse views are essentially diagonal transverse views of the eye. Similar to vertical transverse views, the marker is always positioned at the superior side. Since these are not used in the book, please refer to the suggested readings for further discussion of oblique views.

TIP

In horizontal axial and transverse views, the marker is always positioned at the nasal side.

Mnemonic: HORN FOR HORIZONTAL NASAL.

TIP

In vertical axial and transverse views, the marker is always positioned at the superior side.

Mnemonic: VERS for VERTICAL SUPERIOR.

Longitudinal Views

Longitudinal views provide an anterior–posterior sweep of a specific meridian of the fundus. Like radial views (anterior ocular segment imaging) and transverse views (posterior ocular segment imaging), there are as many longitudinal views as there are hours in a clock. In this view, the tip of the probe is placed on the sclera next to the cornea pointing toward the opposite side of the eye. Here, the marker is always positioned toward the limbus. Thus, the top of the scan is the anterior peripheral side, while the bottom is the posterior side close to the optic nerve. Figure 1-16 illustrates how a longitudinal view of the 12 o'clock meridian is taken in the right eye.

Figure 1-16 Longitudinal View of the 12 o'clock Meridian (Right Eye)

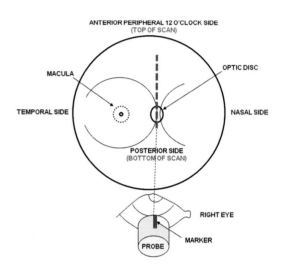

Figure 1-17 illustrates how a longitudinal view of the 9 o'clock meridian is obtained in the right eye.

Figure 1-17 Longitudinal View of the 9 o'clock Meridian (Right Eye)

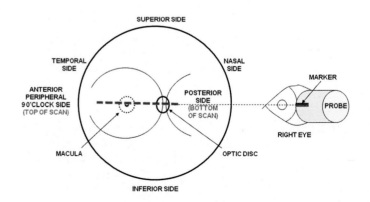

Finally, one can shift the probe away from the limbus to obtain a more peripheral longitudinal view of a particular meridian of the fundus. Figure 1-18 shows how a peripheral longitudinal view of the 9 o'clock meridian is recorded in the right eye.

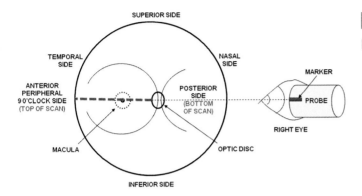

Figure 1-18 Peripheral Longitudinal View of the 9 o'clock Meridian (Right Eye)

TIP

In longitudinal views, the marker is always positioned toward the limbus.

Mnemonic: LOLI for LONGITUDINAL LIMBUS.

For further information on B-scan ultrasound probe orientations, please refer to the suggested readings on ultrasonography found at the end of the atlas.

FORMAT OF THE VIDEO ATLAS

Each case is presented with a UBM or B-scan ultrasound image, as well as a diagnosis. Information about how each scan is obtained (its view) is likewise indicated. Note that the ultrasound findings are properly labeled for ease of identification.

Each case comes with a video clip on the companion Web site, numbered according to the Appendix: List of Videos found at the end of the book. To appreciate the motion of ophthalmic tissues described in each case, one should observe its corresponding video on the Web site. Instructions for accessing the Web site are provided on the inside front cover of the book.

When viewing ultrasound images in the video atlas, bear in mind that the video scans were obtained with patients in a reclined position facing up, unless otherwise indicated. Hence, the right side of the scan is always the dependent portion of the eye.

The following abbreviations are used throughout the video atlas:

VH—Vitreous Hemorrhage
PVD—Posterior Vitreous Detachment
RD—Retinal Detachment
TRD—Traction Retinal Detachment
CD—Choroidal Detachment

Definition of terms used to characterize aftermovement in the video atlas:

jiggle—to move with little jerks
shake—to move irregularly to and fro
undulate—to move in a wavy, sinuous, and flowing manner

SECTION II

Forms of Ophthalmic Ultrasound Movement

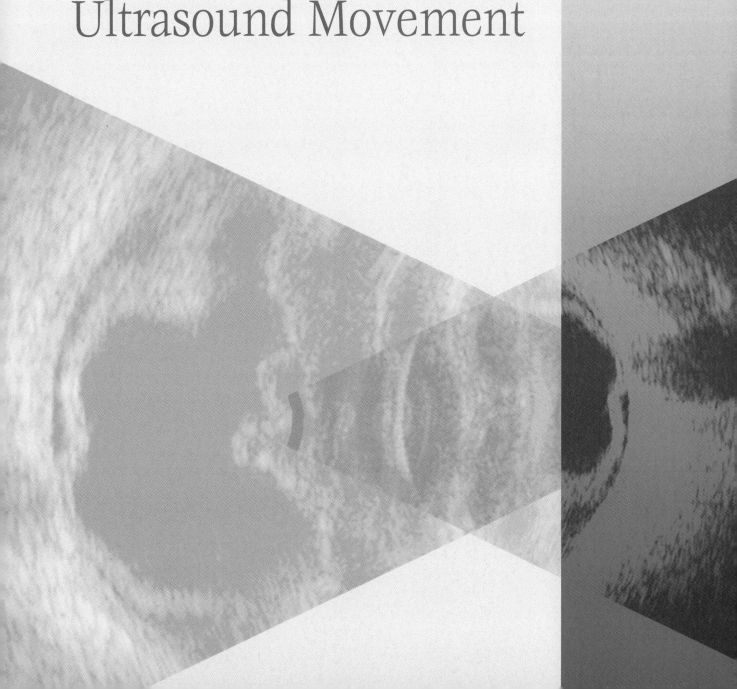

Convection

2

For many years now, dynamic ultrasonography has been considered to be an important adjunct to both two-dimensional (2D) and three-dimensional (3D) B-scan imaging. It brings the element of motion within the realm of digital image capture, playback, storage, retrieval, and analysis.[2] As a result, dynamic 2D B-scan recording of ocular pathologies can simply be reviewed by others in the ophthalmic team, even in the absence of the patient, for the purpose of diagnostic verification or surgical planning.

Dynamic ultrasonography vividly captures the three basic forms of movement described in literature: convection, aftermovement, and vascularity. In addition, two other types of motion have been observed in the eye: gravity-dependent and reflex movements.[3] These types of motion shall be presented and discussed in the following order: convection, gravity-dependent movement, reflex motion, vascularity, and aftermovement.

CONVECTION

Convection is defined as slow, spontaneous motion representing convection currents of fine particles within a cavity. To generate this type of movement, the probe is held steady on the globe, while the patient's eye is fixed in a particular direction of gaze during video recording.

Figure 2-1 Vitreous Hemorrhage in Diabetic Retinopathy

Transverse View

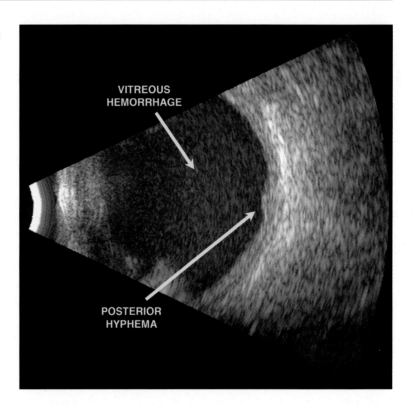

VITREOUS HEMORRHAGE

POSTERIOR HYPHEMA

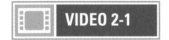

Convection may be observed in long-standing vitreous hemorrhage, where the consistency of the vitreous gel has undergone considerable syneresis and liquefaction. This is a diabetic eye with vitreous hemorrhage. Blood has settled on the retinal surface, termed posterior hyphema. Observe the convection of blood in the vitreous.

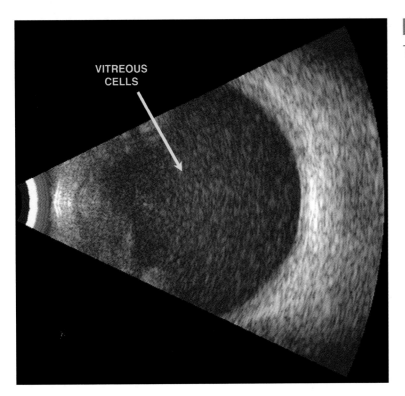

VITREOUS CELLS

Figure 2-2 Vitreous Cells in Endophthalmitis
Transverse View

In this eye with endophthalmitis, the vitreous is also filled with cells that constantly swirl around. Note that based on convection alone, one can hardly distinguish vitreous hemorrhage from endophthalmitis. Hence, a good clinical history should be relied upon.

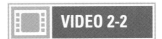

VIDEO 2-2

TIP

Vitreous hemorrhage and endophthalmitis can hardly be differentiated by ultrasound alone.

Figure 2-3 Vitreous Debris

Horizontal Axial View

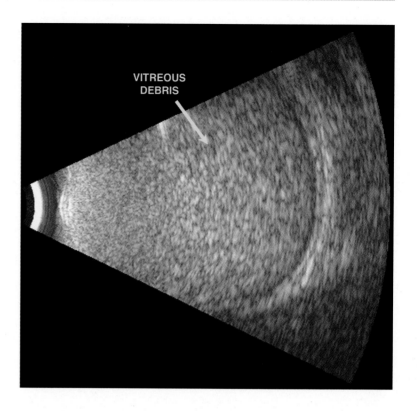

VITREOUS
DEBRIS

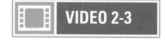

This eye is filled with vitreous particles that are in constant motion, but its etiology is not clear from the clinical history. In the absence of any helpful information, eyes presenting this way are labeled as vitreous debris.

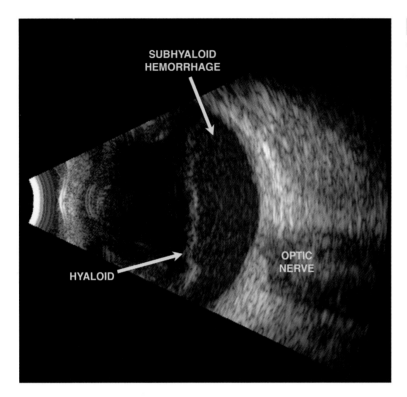

Figure 2-4 Hemorrhagic Complete Posterior Vitreous Detachment

Horizontal Axial View

This scan depicts a complete posterior vitreous detachment associated with subhyaloid hemorrhage (see Chapter 7). Here, blood that is present beneath the hyaloid displays a convection type of movement.

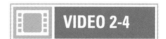

Figure 2-5 Hemorrhagic Closed-Funnel Retinal Detachment and Functioning Glaucoma Implant

Peripheral Transverse View

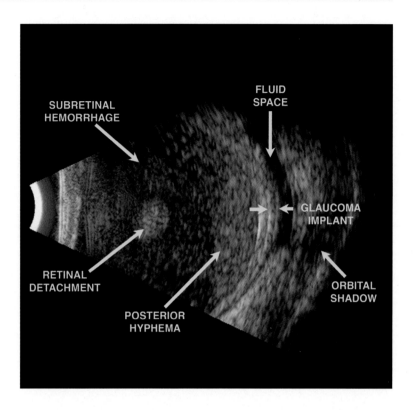

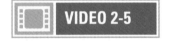

This case has a hemorrhagic type of closed-funnel retinal detachment (see Chapter 8). On transverse scan, the cross section of the closed retinal funnel appears solid and circular. In this eye, subretinal blood is set in constant motion even when the eye remains still. Note the presence of a glaucoma drainage implant (opposing arrows) next to the scleral wall that shadows the orbit. This device appears to be functioning based on the presence of an echolucent fluid space over the implant.

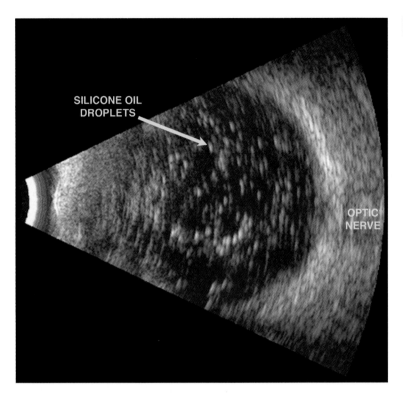

Figure 2-6 Silicone Oil Droplets

Horizontal Axial View

Following silicone oil removal, tiny droplets of the material may remain dispersed in the eye exhibiting streaks of bright, point-like floaters in the vitreous. Observe the convection of silicone oil droplets in this eye.

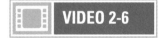

VIDEO 2-6

Figure 2-7 Silicone Oil Droplets

Horizontal Axial View

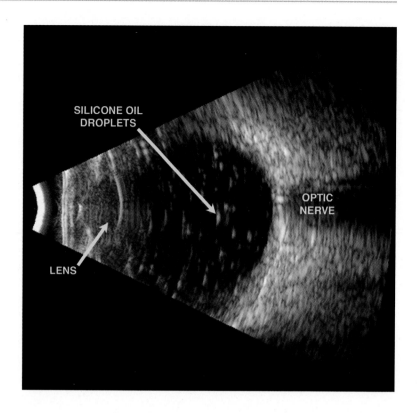

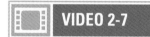

This other case shows remnants of silicone oil in the vitreous, to a lesser degree than the preceding example. It also demonstrates a convection type of movement.

Gravity-Dependent Movement

3

Gravity-dependent movement is motion observed in the eye or orbit that follows the law of gravity. To generate this type of movement, the probe is positioned on the eye during video acquisition as it is made to look from side to side along the axis of the marker or as the head is shifted from a dependent to a nondependent position, and vice versa.

Figure 3-1 Vitreous Hemorrhage from Neovascularization of the Disc in Diabetic Retinopathy

Horizontal Axial View

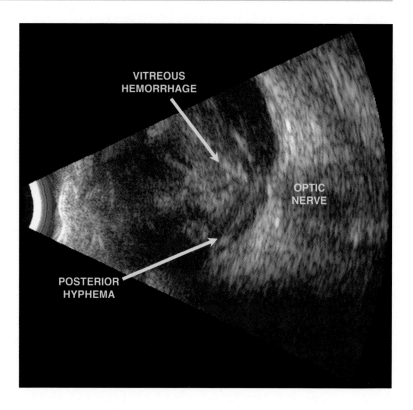

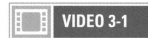

This is a case of diabetic retinopathy, with neovascularization of the disc (NVD) as the source of the vitreous hemorrhage. In this eye, a layer of blood has formed on the surface of the retina, termed posterior hyphema. On dynamic examination, this layer is noted to shift to a more dependent part of the eye.

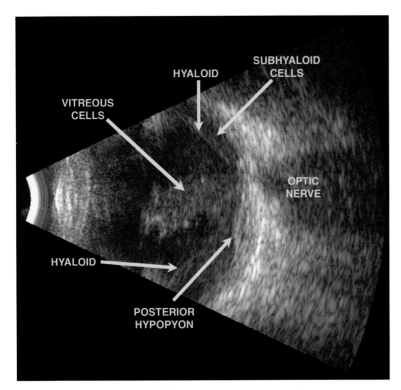

Figure 3-2 Exudative V-Shaped Posterior Vitreous Detachment in Endophthalmitis
Horizontal Axial View

This eye, on the other hand, is filled with vitreous and subhyaloid cells from severe endophthalmitis. Like the previous case, a layer of inflammatory cells has settled on the retinal surface, termed posterior hypopyon. Again, this layer moves against the direction of eye gaze and follows the law of gravity. Note that the vitreous and the wide, V-shaped posterior vitreous detachment shake a bit as the eye moves back and forth (see Chapters 6 and 7).

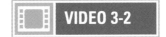

Figure 3-3 Posterior Lens Dislocation with Vitreous Hemorrhage

Horizontal Axial View

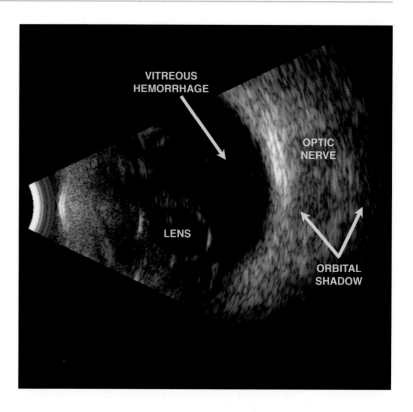

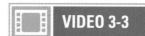

This case shows a dislocated lens that is suspended in the vitreous. It displays a circular outline in an en-face orientation and appears echolucent because of its inherent transparent state. With eye movement, the lens shifts to a more dependent part of the eye while the vitreous undulates (see Chapter 6). Additionally, it casts a shadow on the orbit.

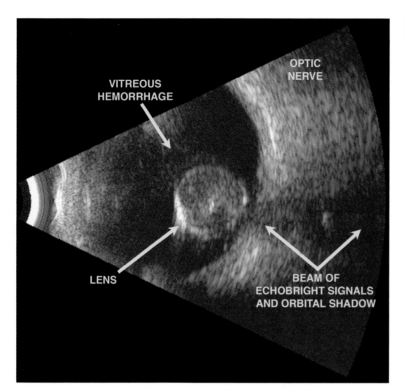

Figure 3-4 Posterior Lens Dislocation with Vitreous Hemorrhage
Vertical Axial View

This eye presents with a dislocated cataractous lens floating in the vitreous. In contrast to a normal lens, the cataractous type is much more visible on ultrasound. This coin-like mass typically casts a flared beam of echobright signals and orbital shadow posterior to it, similar to metallic intraocular foreign bodies (see Chapter 7). On dynamic examination, the lens moves against the direction of eye gaze and settles at a more dependent section of the vitreous. Note the undulation of the vitreous gel (see Chapter 6).

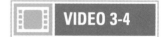

Figure 3-5 Posterior Lens Dislocation with Retinal Detachment

Horizontal Axial View

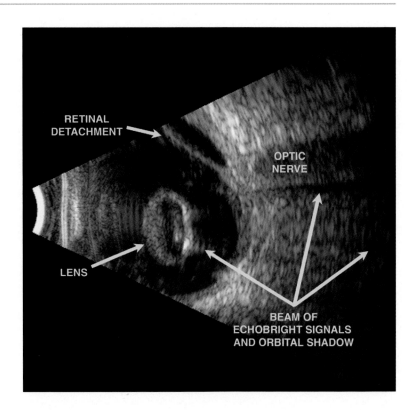

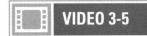

Similarly, this case depicts a dislocated cataractous lens floating in the vitreous, but closer to the posterior pole (temporal or lower half of the scan). Nasal retinal detachment is also present (upper half of the scan). Here, the lens casts a wide beam of echobright signals and orbital shadow to the right of it, blocking the view of the posterior pole. Whenever a situation like this is encountered, one should change the position of the patient's head or that of the probe during dynamic examination, to properly evaluate the macula. Note that the retina shakes a bit as the eye moves (see Chapter 8).

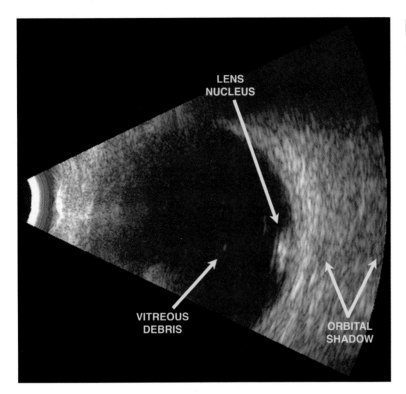

Figure 3-6 Posterior Lens Nucleus Dislocation
Vertical Transverse View

This scan demonstrates a cataractous lens nucleus dislocation, with the nucleus resting on its side on the surface of the retina. This time, the nucleus casts a more subtle shadow on the orbit, similar to that of a normal lens. In this example, the nucleus slides down towards the inferior retina.

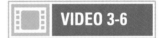

Figure 3-7 Posterior Intraocular Lens
Dislocation
Transverse View

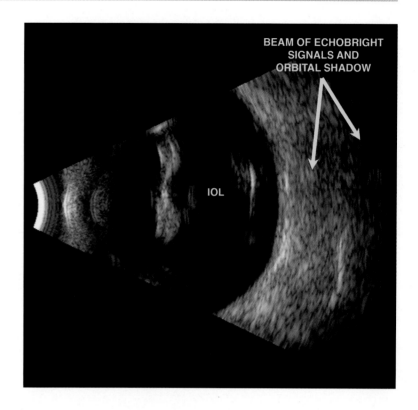

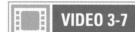

Intraocular lenses (IOLs) are less discernible than cataractous lenses on ultrasound because of the implant's transparent material. Thus, when an IOL becomes dislocated in the vitreous, only parts of its outline become visible at a time. Nonetheless, they still cast a beam of echobright signals and orbital shadow behind them like cataractous lenses. Observe the IOL as, following the law of gravity, it bounces back and forth against the direction of eye movement.

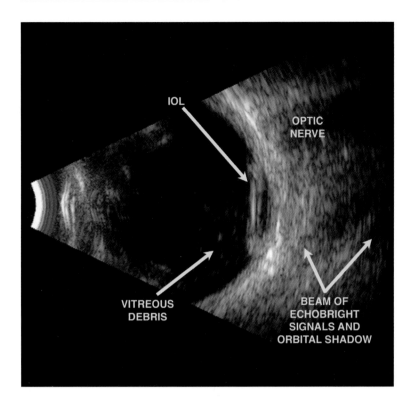

This case also demonstrates an intraocular lens dislocation. Here, the implant is noted to rest on its side on the surface of the retina. Note that whenever the IOL slides toward the surface of the optic nerve, its wide beam of echobright signals and orbital shadow completely masks the optic nerve shadow.

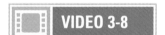

TIP

In posterior cataractous or intraocular lens dislocations, one should always verify the status of the macula because its view may be obstructed by the lens.

Figure 3-9 Orbital Varix

Transverse View

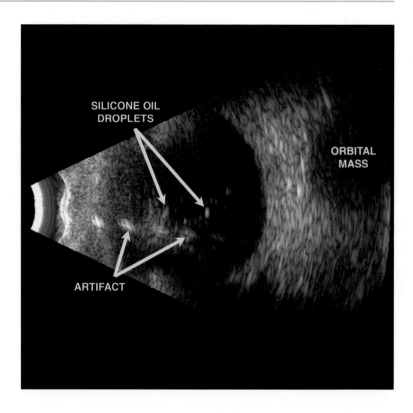

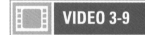

Interestingly, an orbital varix exhibits a unique form of gravity-dependent movement. In this eye, a mass is noted at the posterior orbit when the patient bends his head toward the knees. The mass notably disappears after the patient straightens up. Here, silicone oil remnants are also present in the vitreous.

Reflex Motion

4

Reflex motion refers to the change in the shape of the iris relative to the angle that occurs following exposure to light or dark. To generate reflex motion, the patient is instructed to fix in one particular direction of gaze while the probe is positioned over the angle of interest. Video recording is then started with the room lights on and continued with turning the lights off, or vice versa, eliciting dilation or constriction of the pupil, respectively. This form of motion is generated during ultrasound biomicroscopic tests that are performed for evaluating the angle in eyes suspected of glaucoma.[4]

Figure 4-1 Narrow, Occludable Angle

Radial View

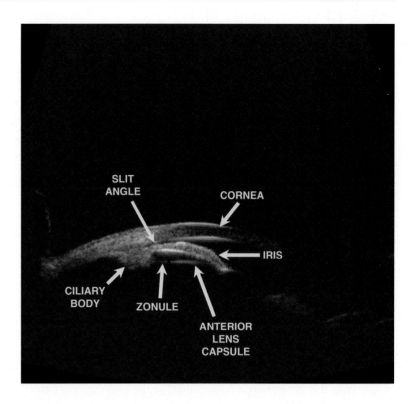

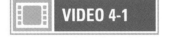

In this case, the angle between the cornea and the iris is narrow or slit-like in a well-lit room. As the light is turned off, the iris shortens during pupillary dilation, and the angle becomes occluded. This is the dynamic picture seen in narrow, occludable angles.

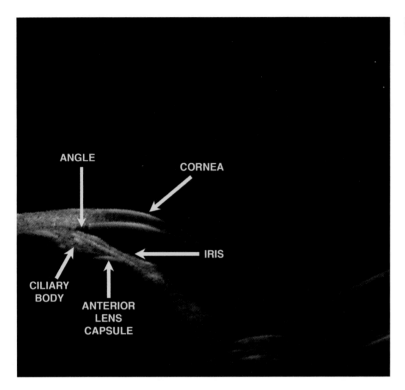

Figure 4-2 Plateau Iris Syndrome
Radial View

Here, the angle is open with the room lights on. When the room is darkened, the iris shortens with pupillary dilation, and the angle becomes occluded. Note that the anterior part of the ciliary body is abnormally positioned beneath the iris. This is believed to push the iris against the angle, further crowding it. This is the configuration of the angle observed in plateau iris syndrome.

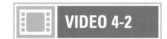

Figure 4-3 Pigment Dispersion Syndrome

Radial View

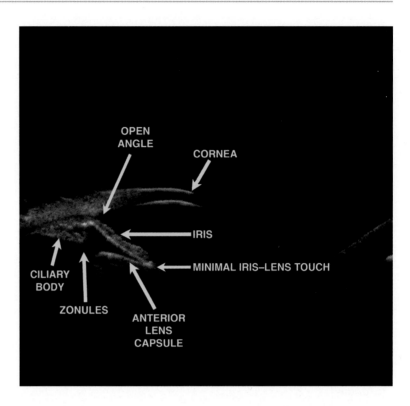

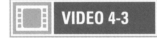

This eye, on the other hand, shows a wide-open angle in a dark room with minimal iris–lens touch. As the light is turned on, the iris lengthens with pupillary constriction, and sags toward the surface of the lens (sagging iris profile). This exaggerates the iris–lens contact, which is believed to cause rubbing between the posterior iris surface and the anterior zonules present at the lens periphery. Consequently, iris pigments are released that eventually get deposited at the angle. This is the profile of the iris depicted in pigment dispersion syndrome.

Vascularity

5

Vascularity refers to rapid, spontaneous motion that signifies blood flow within vessels. To generate vascularity, the patient keeps the eye fixed in a particular direction. Once the area that exhibits blood flow is in view, the probe is held in that position and video recording is obtained.

There are two forms of vascularity observed in the eye: external vascularity, which may be depicted by highly-perfused tissues in the eye, and internal vascularity, which may be demonstrated by ocular and orbital masses.

EXTERNAL VASCULARITY

External vascularity may be observed along portions of the retina and the choroid, both of which have extensive vascular supply. This vascular activity is always subtle in presentation and may be easily missed when one's attention is focused on the more dominant ophthalmic findings.

Figure 5-1 Vitreous Hemorrhage, Serous Partial Posterior Vitreous Detachment, and Hemorrhagic Retinal Detachment

Transverse View

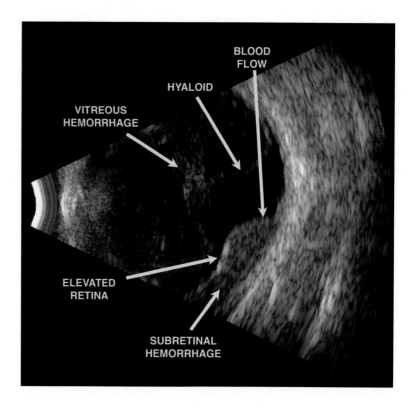

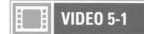

In the case above, vitreous hemorrhage is present and the retina is elevated by subretinal accumulation of blood. Partial serous posterior vitreous detachment is likewise present. On dynamic examination, rapid blood flow takes place along the retinal detachment, while the vitreous and the partially detached hyaloid demonstrate a wave-like aftermovement (see Chapter 6 and 7). Note the shifting motion of the retinal detachment and subretinal blood.

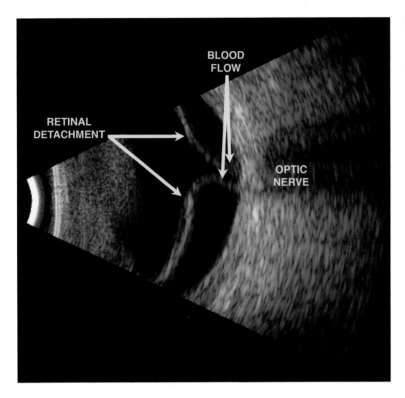

Figure 5-2 Serous Open-Funnel Retinal Detachment
Horizontal Axial View

External vascularity is also demonstrated in this case of serous open-funnel retinal detachment (see Chapter 8). Although not usually seen in retinal detachments, rapid blood flow in this eye can be observed along both sides of the retinal funnel close to the surface of the optic nerve.

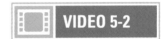

VIDEO 5-2

Figure 5-3 Serous Choroidal Detachment

Transverse View

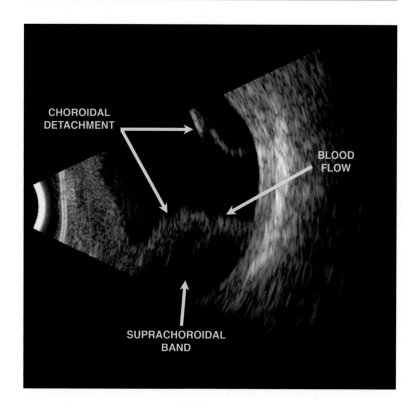

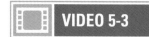

Above is a transverse scan that shows a bilobed, serous choroidal detachment (see Chapter 9). At first glance, rapid blood flow appears to come from the choroid. On closer examination, however, it can be observed to actually take place along the retinal surface. In this eye, a suprachoroidal band is visible within the lower choroidal detachment, which could be a vortex vein, a ciliary vessel, or a ciliary nerve.[1]

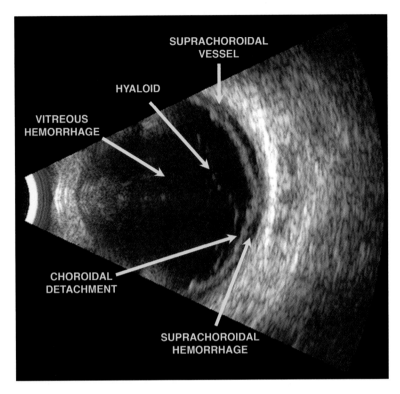

This eye displays vitreous hemorrhage, partial serous posterior vitreous detachment, and low-lying hemorrhagic CD at the periphery (see Chapters 7 and 9). On dynamic examination, blood flow within the suprachoroidal vessel is rapid but subtle. As the eye moves, watch the wave-like motion of the hyaloid and the jiggly aftermovement of the choroid.

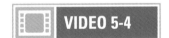

Figure 5-5 Serous Open-Funnel Retinal Detachment and Serous Choroidal Detachment

Horizontal Axial View

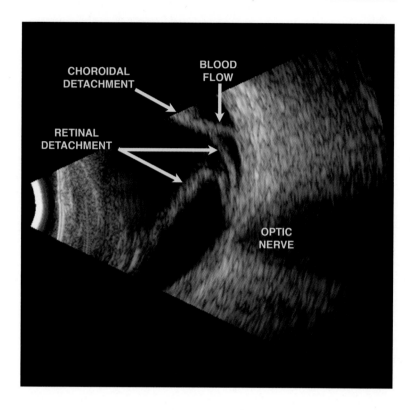

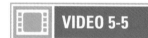

This case presents with both retinal and choroidal detachment (see Chapters 8 and 9). In this eye, blood flow occurs along the choroidal layer.

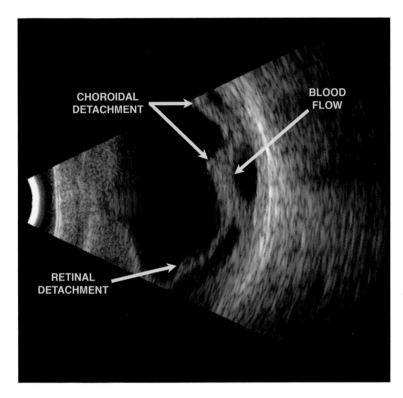

Figure 5-6 Serous Retinal Detachment and Serous Choroidal Detachment

Peripheral Transverse View

This eye shows both low-lying serous retinal detachment and low-lying serous choroidal detachment at the periphery (see Chapters 8 and 9). In this eye, blood flow is observed along the choroid and not the overlying retina.

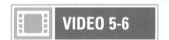

Figure 5-7   Hemorrhagic Kissing Choroidal Detachment

Horizontal Axial View

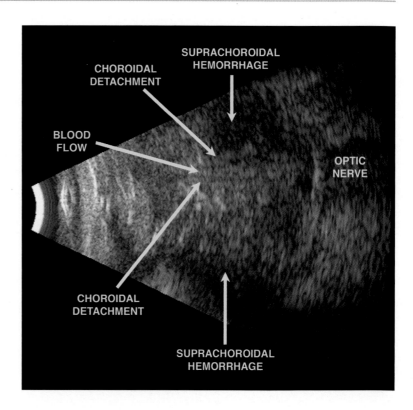

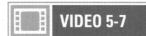

Above is a case that depicts a hemorrhagic, kissing type of choroidal detachment (see Chapter 9). On closer examination, blood can be observed to flow rapidly along the apposed retinal surfaces, sandwiched by the "kissing" choroidal elevation on both sides.

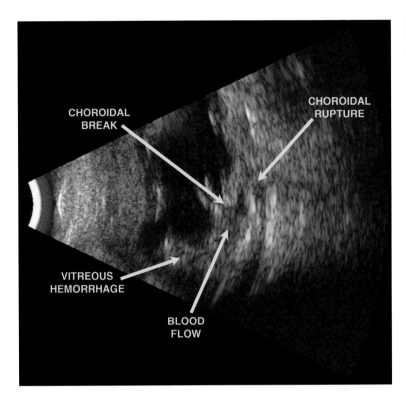

Figure 5-8 Choroidal Rupture

Peripheral Longitudinal View

This eye demonstrates a posttraumatic choroidal rupture at the periphery. On longitudinal scan, the upper edge of the choroidal break can be observed to jut into the vitreous cavity like a faucet. On dynamic examination, choroidal blood is seen to gush from this site toward the vitreous.

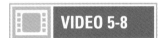

INTERNAL VASCULARITY

Internal vascularity may be observed in tumors, foremost among which are dome-shaped choroidal melanomas. These tumors exhibit a classic shimmering motion within the mass, which arises from a robust internal vascular network.

Figure 5-9 Dome-Shaped Choroidal Melanoma with Hemorrhagic Retinal Detachment

Transverse View

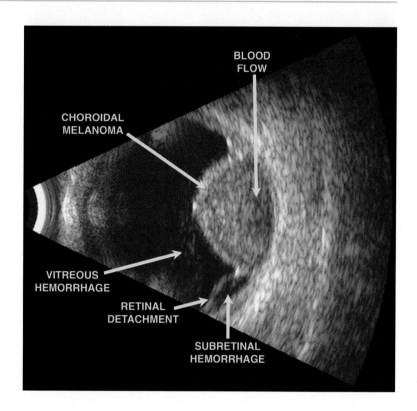

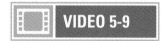 **VIDEO 5-9**

In this case, examine the shimmering pattern of internal vascularity of the choroidal melanoma. Here, vitreous hemorrhage and a hemorrhagic type of retinal detachment are likewise present (see Chapter 8).

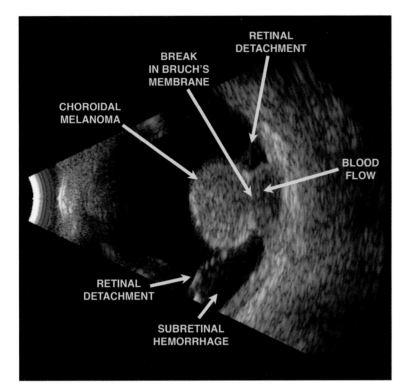

Figure 5-10 Collar-Button Choroidal Melanoma with Hemorrhagic Retinal Detachment

Transverse View

Mushroom-shaped choroidal melanomas result from a break in Bruch's membrane, and these are referred to as collar-button melanomas. In this eye, there is a shimmering type of internal vascularity at the upper half of the mass. Note the secondary hemorrhagic retinal detachment associated with the melanoma (see Chapter 8).

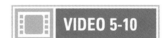

Figure 5-11 Collar-Button Choroidal Melanoma with Hemorrhagic Retinal Detachment

Transverse View

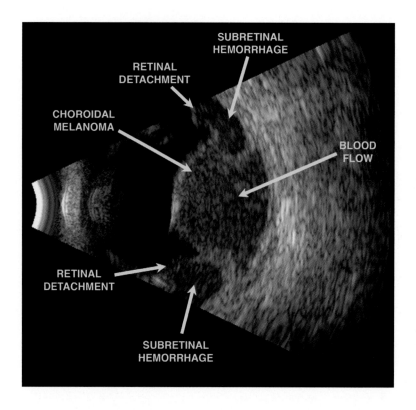

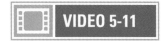

This is another collar-button melanoma associated with hemorrhagic retinal detachment (see Chapter 8). Here, the size of the mass and the break in Bruch's membrane is bigger than the previous case. On dynamic examination, a shimmering motion is visible within the mass.

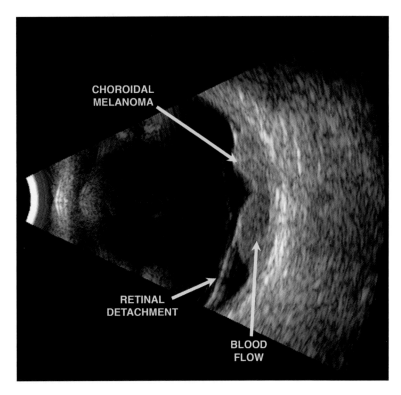

Figure 5-12 Irregular-Shaped Choroidal Melanoma with Serous Retinal Detachment
Transverse View

This case exhibits a choroidal melanoma with a peanut-shaped surface topography. In this eye, a serous type of retinal detachment has formed (see Chapter 8). This mass likewise depicts a shimmering type of internal vascularity.

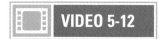

Figure 5-13 Orbital Aneurysm

Transverse View

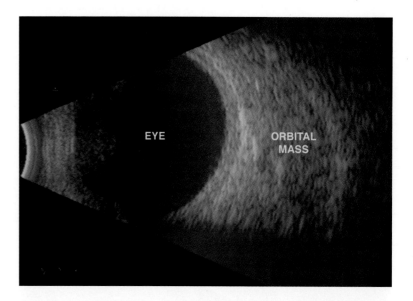

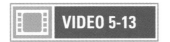

In contrast to the vascular pattern demonstrated in the preceding cases, this orbital aneurysm exhibits a more subtle type of internal vascularity. In this eye, the pear-shaped orbital mass pulsates with the heartbeat.

Aftermovement of the Vitreous

6

Aftermovement is defined as motion following cessation of eye movement. To generate this type of motion, the patient looks from side to side when the marker on the probe is positioned horizontally or up and down when the marker on the probe is positioned vertically during video recording. It is imperative that the probe stay fixed in position as ultrasound recording is obtained to capture the full intraocular motion elicited by the eye movement.

In this section, dynamic ultrasonography demonstrates distinct types of motion inherent to the vitreous, hyaloid, retina, and choroid. It is important to note, however, that motion inherent to a specific tissue may be modified by a host of factors, which makes ultrasound interpretation not only interesting but also challenging to the ultrasound examiner. Thus, a comprehensive knowledge of ocular tissue dynamics is crucial to the differential diagnosis of ocular disease, especially when visual prognosis depends on early surgical intervention.

AFTERMOVEMENT OF THE VITREOUS

The vitreous is normally echolucent. It becomes discernible only when it is set in motion in the presence of vitreous particles. The vitreous classically displays a wave-like, undulating aftermovement. This form of motion is best demonstrated when particles are suspended in the gel-like substance of the vitreous such as calcium soaps in asteroid hyalosis, red blood cells in vitreous hemorrhage, and inflammatory or exudative cells in endophthalmitis, among others.

> **TIP**
>
> The vitreous is normally echolucent. It becomes discernible when it is set in motion in the presence of suspended particles.
>
> **Motion:** wave-like, undulating aftermovement

Figure 6-1 Asteroid Hyalosis

Horizontal Axial View

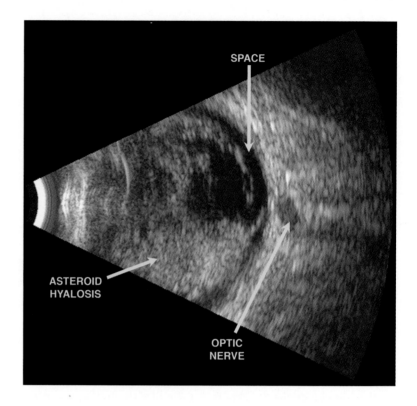

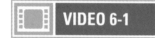

This case depicts asteroid hyalosis. In this condition, calcium soap particles permeate the vitreous gel. On dynamic examination, a space is usually observed between the vitreous particles and the ocular wall, although the vitreous remains adherent to the retinal surface.[1] Observe the undulating aftermovement of the vitreous.

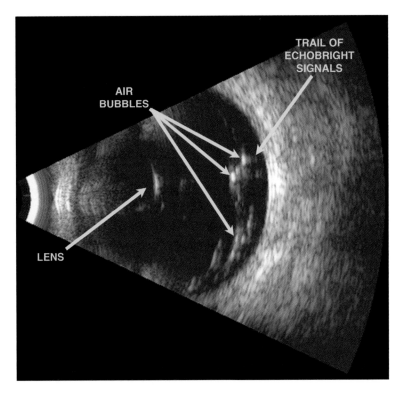

Figure 6-2 Air Bubbles

Transverse View

Following traumatic globe rupture, this eye exhibited a number of bubbles in the vitreous from inadvertent introduction of air. These present as tiny hyperechoic spheres that cast a short trail of echobright signals behind them. With eye movement, they undulate with the vitreous. Because of their echobrightness, air bubbles may be mistaken for metallic intraocular foreign bodies, but the trail of echobright signals generated by air bubbles is unlike those cast by the latter (see Fig. 7-18).

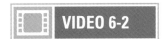

Figure 6-3 Organized Blood Clot

Transverse View

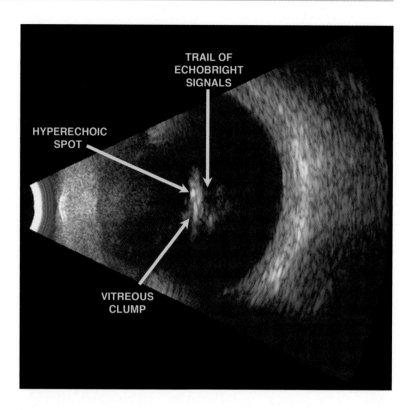

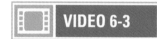

After removal of a glass shard that pierced the eye, this case still showed a hyperechoic spot within the clump of vitreous floating at the center of the eye. Similar to the previous case, this hyperechoic spot may be suspected to be an intraocular foreign body. On dynamic examination, a short trail of echobright signals comes into view as the vitreous undulates. Note that on subsequent surgery, this vitreous finding was confirmed to be an organized blood clot.

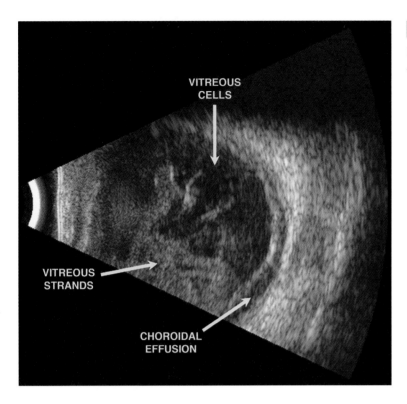

Figure 6-4 Endophthalmitis with Exudative Choroidal Effusion

Transverse View

This eye with endophthalmitis shows vitreous cells and whorl-like strands filling the vitreous cavity. Note that the presence of whorl-like strands in the vitreous is a tell-tale sign of full-blown endophthalmitis. With eye movement, the vitreous undulates. Note the associated exudative type of choroidal effusion in this example.

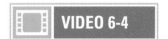

VIDEO 6-4

TIP

The presence of whorl-like strands in the vitreous is a tell-tale sign of full-blown endophthalmitis.

Figure 6-5 Vitreous Debris

Peripheral Transverse View

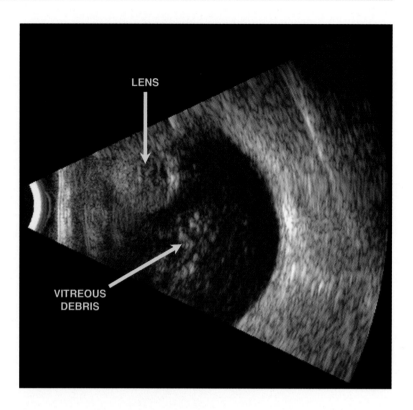

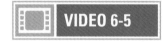

This case presents with vitreous debris. The lens, which is in an en-face orientation on peripheral transverse view, is at its normal location at the anterior vitreous cavity. As the eye moves, the vitreous exhibits a wave-like, undulating aftermovement.

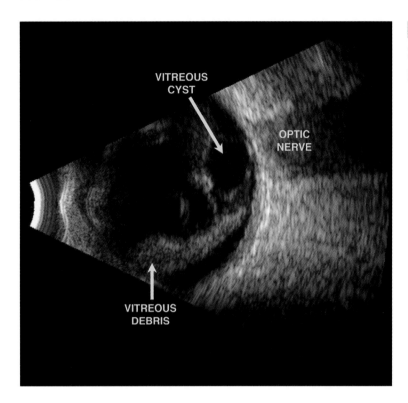

Figure 6-6 Vitreous Debris with Cyst and Serous Partial Posterior Vitreous Detachment
Horizontal Axial View

The vitreous may undergo a cystic type of degeneration, forming a vitreous cyst. In this example, the eye is filled with vitreous debris. Partial serous posterior vitreous detachment is likewise present (see Chapter 7). Observe the slight undulation of the vitreous and hyaloid.

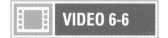

Figure 6-7 Vitreous Hemorrhage

Horizontal Axial View

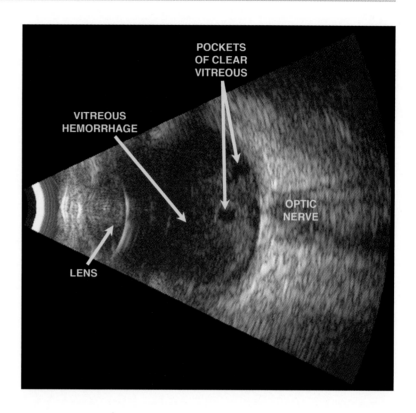

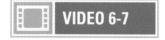

Blood permeates the vitreous in an eye with vitreous hemorrhage. In contrast to the previous case, the cyst-like spaces here are actually pockets of clear vitreous. Here, the vitreous aftermovement is classically wave-like and undulating.

Whenever one encounters a case of vitreous hemorrhage, one should always look for a possible source. Vitreous hemorrhage may result from a small vessel break arising from vitreoretinal traction, a retinal flap tear, choroidal rupture, or neovascularization from diabetic or sickle cell retinopathy, to name a few.

Vitreoretinal Traction usually appears as an echobright spot at the peripheral fundus, with blood coming from it and cascading toward the vitreous.

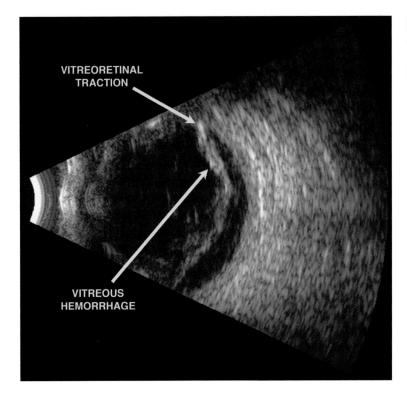

Figure 6-8 Vitreous Hemorrhage from Vitreoretinal Traction

Peripheral Longitudinal View

This case best illustrates vitreous hemorrhage from vitreoretinal traction. Observe the slight vitreous undulation on dynamic examination. It is important to note that cascading images of blood in the vitreous are only demonstrable using longitudinal B-scan views.

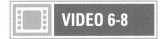

Figure 6-9   Vitreous Hemorrhage from Vitreoretinal Traction

Peripheral Longitudinal View

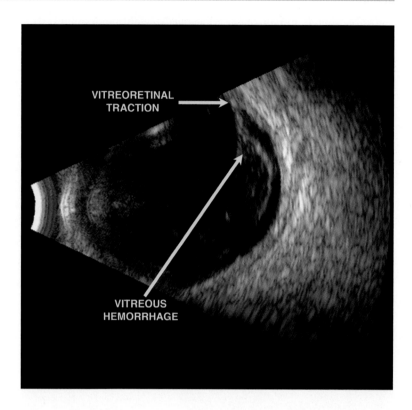

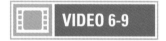

This is another case of vitreous hemorrhage due to vitreoretinal traction, with blood cascading from an echobright spot of vitreoretinal traction at the fundus periphery. Here, the aftermovement of the vitreous is undulating.

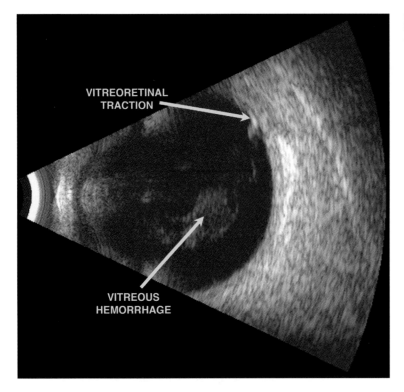

Figure 6-10 Vitreous Hemorrhage from Vitreoretinal Traction

Peripheral Longitudinal View

This eye with vitreous hemorrhage from vitreoretinal traction does not show the cascading pattern as well as the first two cases, but the echobright spot of vitreoretinal traction is remarkably distinct. Again, the vitreous displays a wave-like, undulating aftermovement.

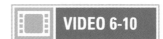 **VIDEO 6-10**

Figure 6-11 Vitreous Hemorrhage from Vitreoretinal Traction

Peripheral Transverse View

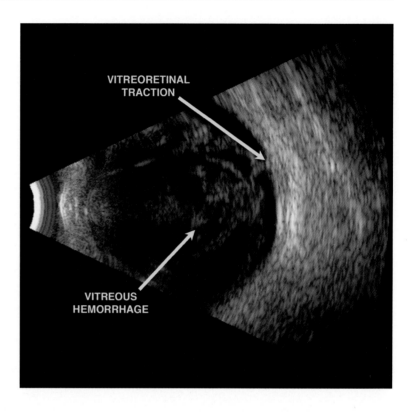

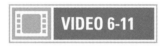

This is another case of vitreous hemorrhage from vitreoretinal traction. Observe that on transverse view, the cascading pattern is no longer depicted. Nevertheless, vitreous aftermovement is wave-like and undulating.

TIP

On longitudinal views, vitreoretinal traction presents as an echobright spot at the retinal periphery, with blood cascading from it toward the vitreous.

One should differentiate vitreous hemorrhage caused by vitreoretinal traction from those resulting from actual retinal flap tears. This is because tears may eventually lead to a full-blown retinal detachment if left undetected. Again, one should obtain longitudinal—not transverse—scans in searching for retinal flap tears.

Retinal Flap Tears are mostly located superiorly. Unlike vitreoretinal traction, a retinal flap tear usually presents as a short, echobright tuft at the peripheral fundus, with an echobright stump next to it or close by on the ocular wall that represents the other edge of the tear.

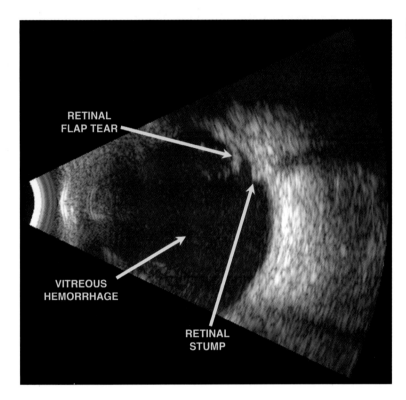

Figure 6-12 Vitreous Hemorrhage from Retinal Flap Tear

Peripheral Longitudinal View

This case presents vitreous hemorrhage resulting from a retinal flap tear. In this eye, both the retinal flap and its stump are shown at the fundus periphery. Observe the wave-like aftermovement of the retinal flap and the vitreous, both of which are still attached to each other.

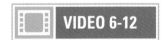

Figure 6-13 Vitreous Hemorrhage from Retinal Flap Tear

Peripheral Longitudinal View

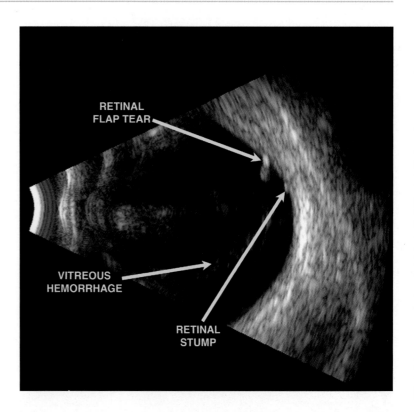

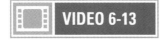

This is another eye with vitreous hemorrhage from a retinal flap tear. This case also presents an echobright tuft at the peripheral fundus. However, the stump of the tear is not as apparent as in the previous example. With eye movement, the retinal flap undulates with the vitreous.

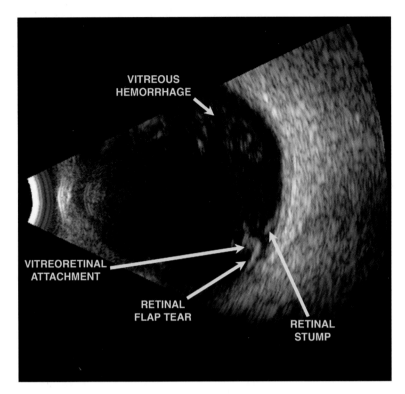

Figure 6-14 Vitreous Hemorrhage from Retinal Flap Tear

Peripheral Longitudinal View

Retinal flap tears do not always occur at the periphery. This particular tear was identified closer to the equator. On dynamic examination, both the echobright retinal tuft and its stump undulate with the vitreous.

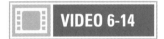

Figure 6-15 Vitreous Hemorrhage from Retinal Flap Tear with Focal Retinal Detachment

Peripheral Longitudinal View

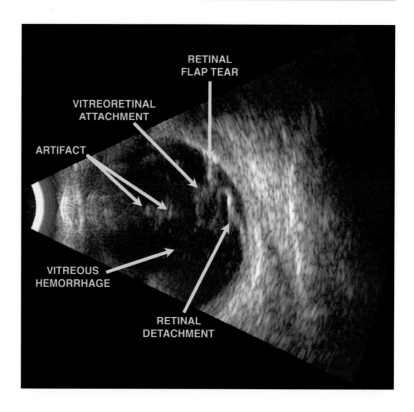

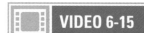

This case of vitreous hemorrhage from retinal flap tear is associated with focal retinal detachment. It shows an echobright retinal tuft at the periphery, with its stump detached to some extent from the ocular wall. Note that the vitreous undulates a bit, while the string-like retina shakes minimally (see Chapter 8).

TIP

On longitudinal views, a retinal flap tear presents as a short, echobright tuft protruding from the peripheral fundus, with blood cascading from it toward the vitreous. More importantly, there is also an echobright stump next to it, representing the other edge of the tear.

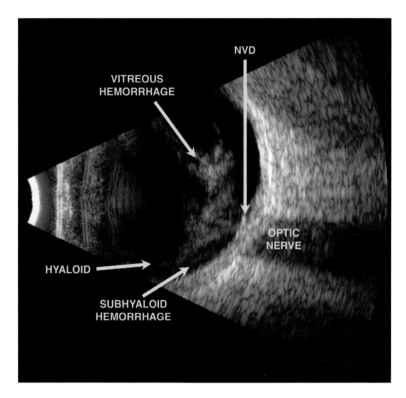

Figure 6-16 Vitreous Hemorrhage from Neovascularization of the Disc and Hemorrhagic Partial Posterior Vitreous Detachment in Diabetic Retinopathy
Horizontal Axial View

Aside from vitreoretinal tractions and retinal flap tears, vitreous hemorrhage may also be secondary to neovascularization of the disc (NVD) in diabetic retinopathy. In this eye, there is seepage of blood beneath the indiscernible hyaloid, leading to partial hemorrhagic posterior vitreous detachment (see Chapter 7). Note that the thread-like hyaloid is rendered indistinct by the presence of subhyaloid hemorrhage. Here, the vitreous moves in a wave-like, undulating fashion, whereas the hyaloid shakes a bit.

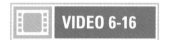

Figure 6-17 Vitreous Hemorrhage from Neovascularization Elsewhere and Hemorrhagic Partial Posterior Vitreous Detachment in Diabetic Retinopathy

Peripheral Transverse View

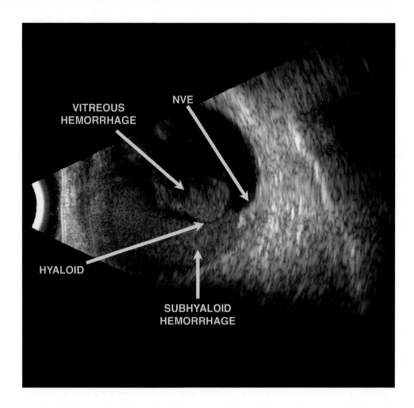

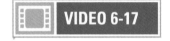

VH may likewise be secondary to neovascularization elsewhere (NVE) in diabetic retinopathy. In this eye, blood has accumulated mostly in the subhyaloid compartment, with partial hemorrhagic posterior vitreous detachment (see Chapter 7). Again the hyaloid is made indiscernible because of the subhyaloid hemorrhage. On dynamic examination, the thread-like hyaloid, as well as blood in both vitreous and subhyaloid compartments, typically undulate.

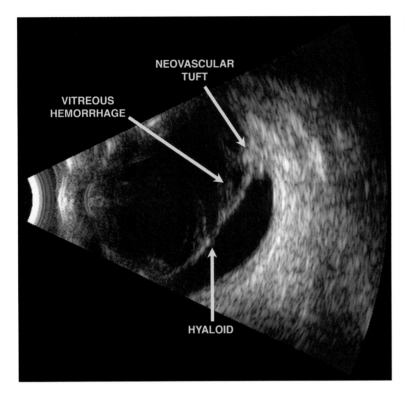

Figure 6-18 Vitreous Hemorrhage and Serous Partial Posterior Vitreous Detachment from Sickle Cell Retinopathy

Peripheral Longitudinal View

Furthermore, vitreous hemorrhage may come from a bleeding neovascular tuft, in eyes with sickle cell retinopathy. Note the associated partial serous posterior vitreous detachment (see Chapter 7). In this particular case, the vitreous and the hyaloid undulate as the eye moves about.

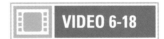

Figure 6-19 Vitreous Hemorrhage, Serous Partial Posterior Vitreous Detachment, and Hemorrhagic Choroidal Effusion from Choroidal Rupture

Peripheral Transverse View

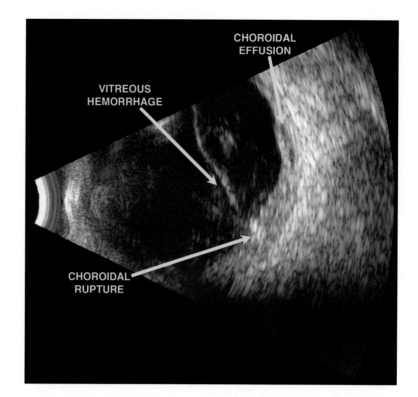

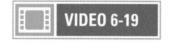

Trauma may be another source of vitreous hemorrhage, as depicted in this eye with vitreous hemorrhage, partial serous posterior vitreous detachment, and hemorrhagic choroidal effusion from choroidal rupture. With movement, both the vitreous and hyaloid undulate. Here, the hyaloid appears to be irregularly thickened owing to the presence of blood in front of the hyaloid (see Chapter 7). Notice the rapid flow of blood along the upper half of the hemorrhagic choroidal effusion.

TIP

Whenever vitreous hemorrhage is encountered, one should always attempt to look for its source.

Aftermovement of the Hyaloid

7

Echographically, the hyaloid surrounding the vitreous is normally thread-like when detached from the retinal surface. It moves with the vitreous, but its aftermovement depends on its extent of separation from the ocular wall. Clinically termed posterior vitreous detachment (PVD), hyaloid detachments may range from partial to complete detachments.

In a majority of cases, hyaloid motion exhibits a wave-like, undulating aftermovement that follows the dynamic behavior of the vitreous. Occasionally, it may be shaky or jiggly, or it may show no aftermovement.

In this section, we shall look at partial PVD, V-shaped PVD, complete PVD, and vitreoschisis.

TIP

When detached, the hyaloid is typically thread-like on ultrasound.

Majority: wave-like, undulating aftermovement
Others: shaky, jiggly, no aftermovement

PARTIAL POSTERIOR VITREOUS DETACHMENTS

In partial PVD, parts of the hyaloid remain attached to the inner surface of the eye.

Figure 7-1 Serous Partial Posterior Vitreous Detachment and Nonfunctioning Glaucoma Implant

Transverse View

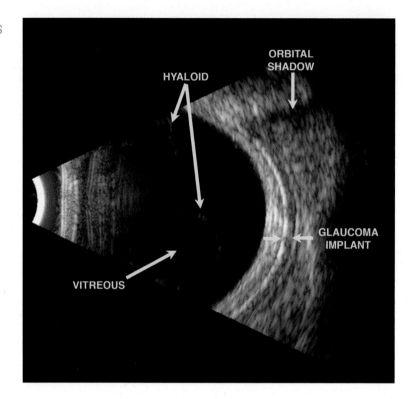

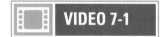

This case shows partial serous posterior vitreous detachment anterior to the equator. Observe how thread-like the hyaloid appears to be. On dynamic examination, the hyaloid and the indiscernible vitreous display a wave-like, undulating aftermovement. In this example, a glaucoma drainage implant (opposing arrows) is also seen hugging the outer surface of the globe, partially shadowing the orbit. This device appears to be nonfunctioning based on the absence of an echolucent fluid space over the implant (see Fig. 2-5).

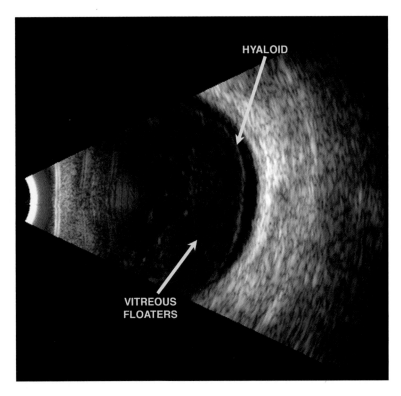

Figure 7-2 Serous Partial Posterior Vitreous Detachment with Vitreous Floaters

Transverse View

This case likewise demonstrates partial serous posterior vitreous detachment involving the periphery. Fine floaters are also present in the vitreous. As the eye moves, both the thread-like hyaloid and the vitreous undulate.

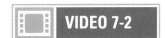

VIDEO 7-2

Figure 7-3 Serous Partial Posterior Vitreous Detachment in Chronic Uveitis

Horizontal Axial View

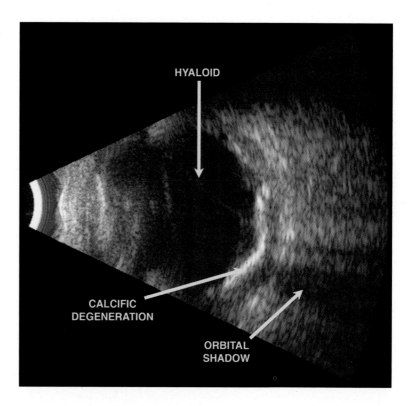

HYALOID

CALCIFIC DEGENERATION

ORBITAL SHADOW

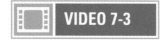

VIDEO 7-3

This eye with previous bouts of posterior uveitis shows partial serous posterior vitreous detachment, with residual attachment to the temporal equator where calcific degeneration has set in (lower half of the scan). Note the orbital shadowing cast by the calcified wall. Upon eye movement, a thickened preretinal membrane can be seen lining the retinal surface in the vicinity of the optic nerve. Additionally, the rest of the hyaloid is detached, but no observable aftermovement can be appreciated.

As more cellular particles accumulate in the vitreous, the hyaloid becomes more distinct and string-like.

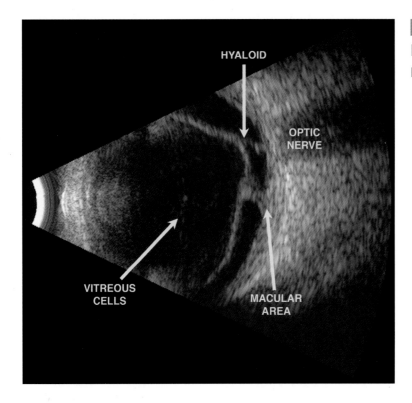

Figure 7-4 Serous Partial Posterior Vitreous Detachment in Chronic Posterior Uveitis

Horizontal Axial View

This eye with chronic posterior uveitis depicts partial serous posterior vitreous detachment, with inflammatory cells permeating the vitreous. Note how much thicker and retina-like the hyaloid has become, compared to the previous case (see Chapter 8). With eye movement, the vitreous and hyaloid typically undulate. Note that the hyaloid remains attached to the surface of the optic nerve and the macula in this example.

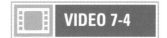

VIDEO 7-4

Hyaloid detachments that are peripheral in location may also appear thick and retina-like in the presence of vitreous particles. Hence, it is important to rule out retinal detachment in such eyes.

Figure 7-5 Serous Partial Posterior Vitreous Detachment and Exudative Choroidal Effusion in Endophthalmitis

Peripheral Transverse View

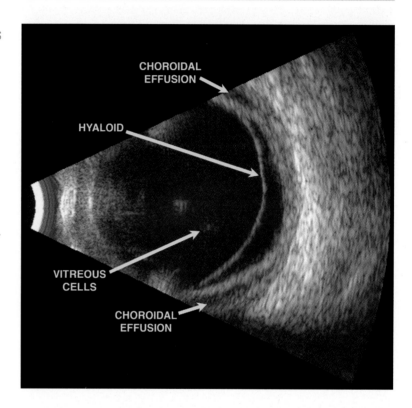

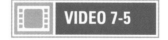

This case of endophthalmitis reveals a peripheral, partial serous posterior vitreous detachment that resembles the retina. However, the eye movement propagates a wave of undulating motion, which is a hyaloid tissue behavior. Note the associated exudative choroidal effusion in this eye.

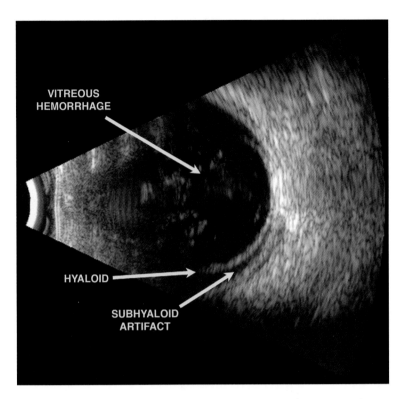

VITREOUS
HEMORRHAGE

HYALOID

SUBHYALOID
ARTIFACT

Figure 7-6 Serous Partial Posterior Vitreous Detachment with Vitreous Hemorrhage

Transverse View

This eye with vitreous hemorrhage also depicts a string-like, partial serous posterior vitreous detachment at the periphery (see Chapter 8). However, the detachment tapers at both ends, which is not characteristic of the retina. With eye movement, the vitreous undulates, but only the lower end of the hyaloid shakes a bit. Note the presence of subhyaloid artifact, which is a form of echographic noise that may be seen beneath minimally detached hyaloids. These minute, fleeting echobright streaks should not be mistaken for actual cellular particles, which have a more speckled appearance.

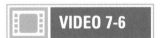
VIDEO 7-6

TIP

The hyaloid becomes distinct and retina-like when the vitreous becomes filled with cellular particles.

V-SHAPED POSTERIOR VITREOUS DETACHMENTS

Of the various forms of PVD presentations, V-shaped hyaloid detachments draw the most clinical attention because of their echographic similarity to funnel-shaped retinal detachments (see Chapter 8). This configuration results from a circumferential separation of the posterior hyaloid, except at the disc or the area over the optic nerve. Such is the profile of the hyaloid in the following case.

Figure 7-7 Serous V-Shaped Posterior Vitreous Detachment with Weiss Ring

Horizontal Axial View

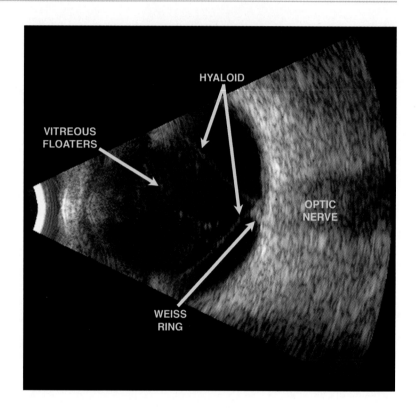

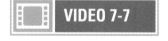 **VIDEO 7-7**

This eye presents with a V-shaped serous posterior vitreous detachment. In this example, the hyaloid is typically thread-like. Note that an echobright elevation can be observed on the surface of the optic nerve. This is called a Weiss ring, the thickest part of the hyaloid that normally surrounds and adheres to the disc.[1] With eye movement, the hyaloid displays a shaky aftermovement.

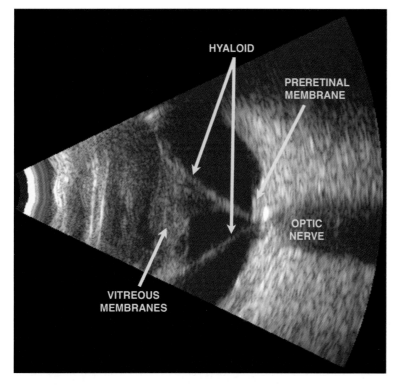

Figure 7-8 Serous V-Shaped Posterior Vitreous Detachment with Vitreous Membranes
Horizontal Axial View

This eye likewise exhibits a V-shaped serous posterior vitreous detachment. Here, observe that the hyaloid is unusually string-like, which is the typical picture of a detached retina (see Chapter 8). Moreover, vitreous membranes are also present. Notice the thickening next to the surface of the optic nerve, which is a preretinal membrane. On dynamic examination, the vitreous and hyaloid typically undulate.

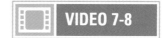

VIDEO 7-8

When cellular particles accumulate in the subhyaloid compartment, the hyaloid becomes echolucent and indistinct. Note that this drop in tissue echobrightness occurs to a lesser extent when cellular particles accumulate beneath retinal detachments (see Chapter 8).

Figure 7-9 Hemorrhagic V-Shaped Posterior Vitreous Detachment

Vertical Axial View

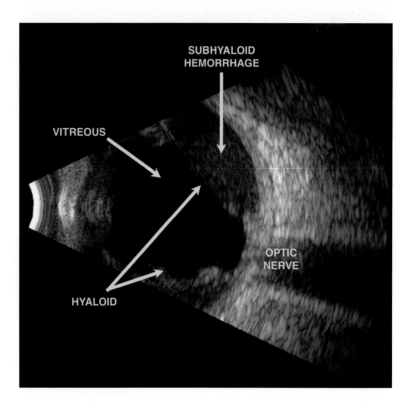

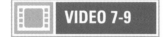 **VIDEO 7-9**

This case illustrates a V-shaped hemorrhagic posterior vitreous detachment that appears to insert along the margins of the optic nerve (see Chapter 8). In this eye, the hyaloid has become echolucent because of the absence of cells in the vitreous and the profusion of cells in the subhyaloid space. As the eye moves, the hyaloid demonstrates an undulating aftermovement.

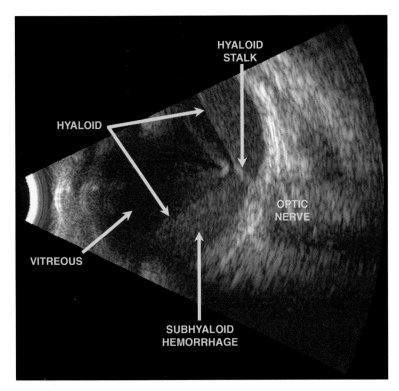

Figure 7-10 Hemorrhagic V-Shaped Posterior Vitreous Detachment with Hyaloid Stalk

Horizontal Axial View

In this eye, the V-shaped hemorrhagic posterior vitreous detachment is almost completely detached, save for a hyaloid stalk that remains connected to the surface of the optic nerve. Notice how, like in the previous case, the hyaloid anterior to the stalk has become imperceptible. On dynamic examination, the hyaloid undulates as subhyaloid blood shifts from side to side.

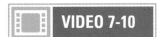

Figure 7-11 Hemorrhagic V-Shaped Posterior Vitreous Detachment with Hyaloid Stalk

Horizontal Axial View

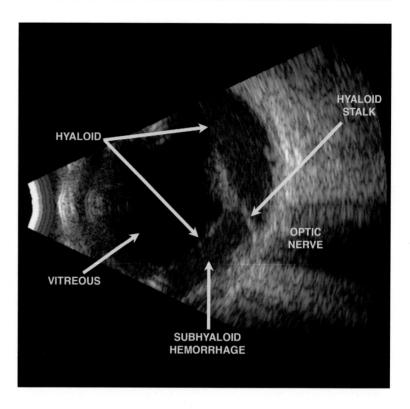

VIDEO 7-11

Similarly, the hyaloid cannot be seen well in this example of hemorrhagic posterior vitreous detachment. Here, a hyaloid stalk is likewise present. With eye movement, the indiscernible hyaloid anterior to the stalk undulates, as the subhyaloid hemorrhage swirls to and fro.

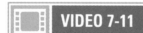

TIP

The hyaloid becomes indiscernible when cellular particles accumulate mainly in the subhyaloid compartment.

With proliferation of hemorrhagic, inflammatory, or tumor cells in both the vitreous and subhyaloid compartments, intraocular changes tend to appear grainier and less defined. Consequently, it becomes more difficult to differentiate the hyaloid from the retina based on their ultrasound appearance. One has to closely observe how the detachment moves during dynamic examination to be able to identify which tissue is involved.

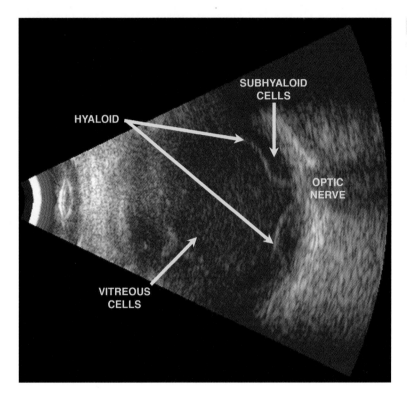

Figure 7-12 Exudative V-Shaped Posterior Vitreous Detachment in Endophthalmitis
Horizontal Axial View

Such is the picture in this case of endophthalmitis, where inflammatory cells have filled the whole eye. In this example, a string-like instead of thread-like, V-shaped exudative posterior vitreous detachment is present (see Chapter 8). However, its aftermovement is distinctly undulating and, as such, attributable to the hyaloid.

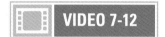

Figure 7-13 Hemorrhagic V-Shaped Posterior Vitreous Detachment with Vitreous Hemorrhage, Hemorrhagic Vitreous Cyst, and Weiss Ring

Horizontal Axial View

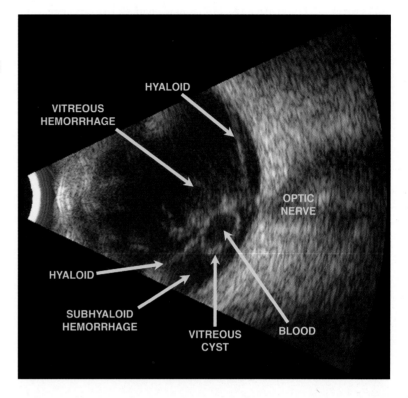

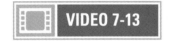

This example displays a V-shaped hemorrhagic posterior vitreous detachment, with a cyst protruding at the temporal side (lower part of the scan). In this eye, blood is present everywhere, including the cyst (hemorrhagic cyst). Note that the hyaloid detachment appears string-like rather than thread-like (see Chapter 8). However, observe that its base is attached directly on the surface of the optic nerve, where a Weiss ring can be seen. Furthermore, dynamic examination points to a hyaloid involvement with its undulating aftermovement.

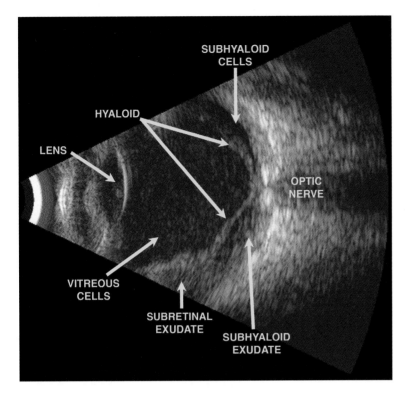

Figure 7-14 Exudative V-Shaped Posterior Vitreous Detachment in Endophthalmitis
Horizontal Axial View

This eye with endophthalmitis exhibits a V-shaped exudative posterior vitreous detachment that resembles a retinal detachment. Here, inflammatory cells are present everywhere. Upon eye movement, its irregular thickness, undulating aftermovement, and fleeting separation from the surface of the optic nerve can only be attributed to the hyaloid. Note the presence of subretinal exudation at the temporal equator (bottom part of the scan).

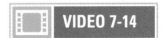 **VIDEO 7-14**

TIP

The hyaloid may resemble the retina when cellular particles accumulate in both vitreous and subhyaloid compartments.

COMPLETE POSTERIOR VITREOUS DETACHMENTS

In complete PVDs, the vitreous totally separates from the retina, allowing the posterior hyaloid to freely undulate with the rest of the vitreous.

Figure 7-15 Serous Complete Posterior Vitreous Detachment in Endophthalmitis

Horizontal Axial View

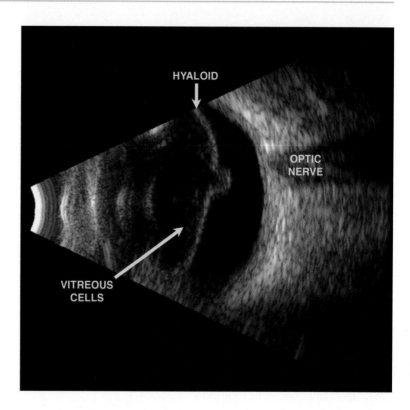

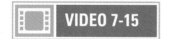 **VIDEO 7-15**

Complete serous posterior vitreous detachment is best demonstrated in this eye with endophthalmitis. On dynamic examination, the hyaloid undulates with the vitreous. Note that the hyaloid appears unusually string-like and similar to the retina because of the presence of cellular particles in front of the hyaloid (see Chapter 8).

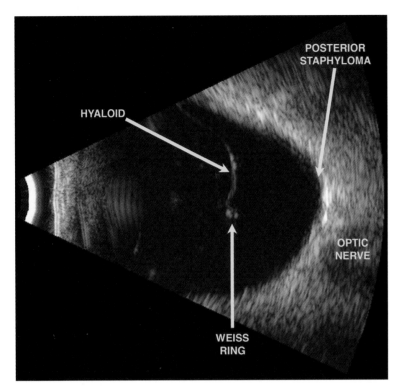

Figure 7-16 Serous Complete Posterior Vitreous Detachment with Weiss Ring in Myopia

Horizontal Axial View

This eye exhibits complete serous posterior vitreous detachment in a myopic globe, as shown by the presence of a posterior staphyloma. Here, the hyaloid is typically thread-like. As the eye moves, both the vitreous and hyaloid undulate, whereas the Weiss ring remains relatively fixed, presumably by an indiscernible strand adherent to the surface of the optic nerve.

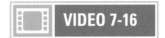

Figure 7-17 Serous Complete Posterior Vitreous Detachment and Posterior Lens Dislocation in Myopia

Horizontal Axial View

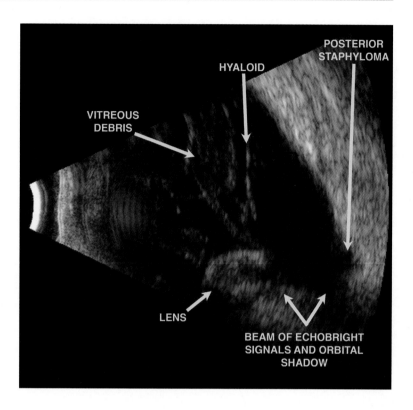

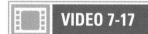

This case also depicts complete serous posterior vitreous detachment in a myopic eye. Here, the thread-like hyaloid is weighed down by a dislocated cataractous lens. In this example, the lens and its beam of echobright signals and orbital shadow shift from side to side (see Chapter 3), while the vitreous and hyaloid undulate before it.

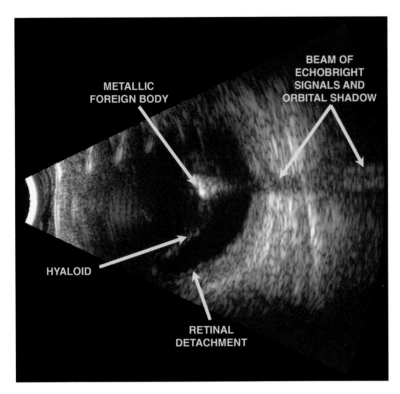

Figure 7-18 Serous Complete Posterior Vitreous Detachment and Low-Lying Retinal Detachment secondary to Metallic Intraocular Foreign Body
Vertical Para-Axial View

Here is another case of complete serous posterior vitreous detachment, with a hyperechoic metallic foreign body stuck to the thread-like hyaloid. With eye movement, the posterior hyaloid undulates. Here, note the flared beam of echobright signals and orbital shadow that is typically cast by metallic foreign bodies posteriorly. A low-lying retinal detachment is also present in this eye (see Chapter 8).

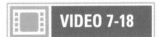

VIDEO 7-18

TIP

Metallic intraocular foreign bodies classically cast a flared beam of echobright signals and orbital shadow behind them.

Figure 7-19 Serous Complete Posterior Vitreous Detachment in Chronic Uveitis

Horizontal Axial View

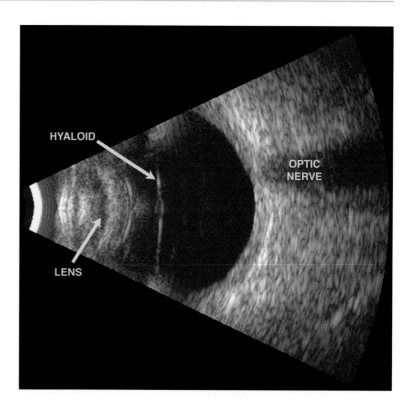

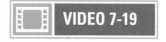

This case illustrates complete serous posterior vitreous detachment after long-standing uveitis. On dynamic examination, the thread-like posterior hyaloid, which is now closer to the lens, displays a shaky type of aftermovement.

VITREOSCHISIS

Vitreoschisis is a condition where the cortical vitreous splits from the hyaloid surface, thereby forming an enclosed space.

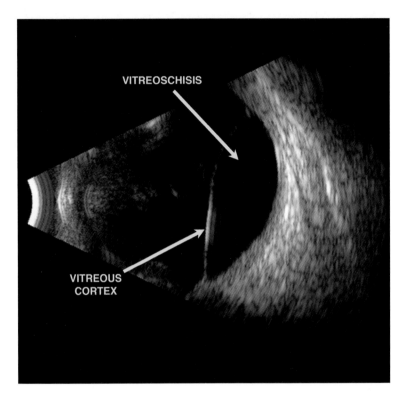

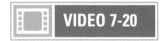

Figure 7-20 Serous Vitreoschisis

Transverse View

In this example, the vitreous cortex appears thin and hair-like on transverse scan. It has a dome-shaped configuration because the hyaloid is still attached to the retinal surface. Here, the aftermovement is jiggly.

VIDEO 7-20

Vitreoschisis exhibits a split-hyaloid picture when the hyaloid has detached from the retinal surface. This presentation is due to the simultaneous imaging of the vitreous cortex and the hyaloid. Whenever this is observed, one should verify that the hyaloid is not merely folded over on itself by correlating dynamic transverse views with longitudinal views.

Figure 7-21 Hemorrhagic Vitreoschisis and Hemorrhagic Partial Posterior Vitreous Detachment

Transverse View

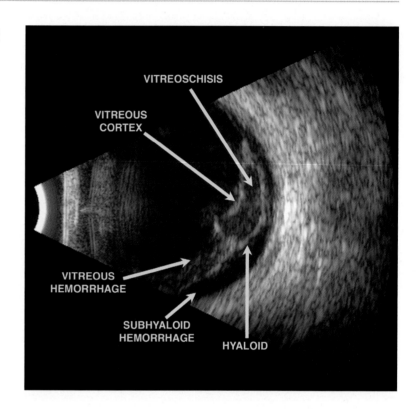

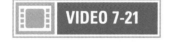

This case presents with vitreous hemorrhage, partial hemorrhagic posterior vitreous detachment, and a split-hyaloid appearance. Note that blood is found within the schisis cavity (hemorrhagic vitreoschisis) and subhyaloid compartments. In this eye, the vitreous cortex undulates more than the hyaloid.

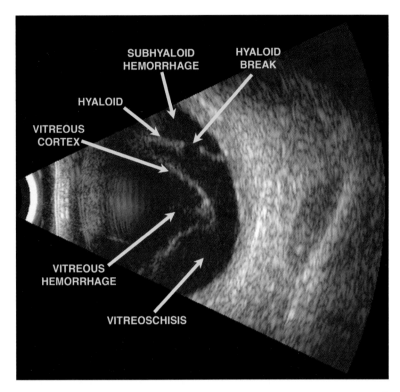

Figure 7-22 Hemorrhagic Vitreoschisis and Hemorrhagic Partial Posterior Vitreous Detachment
Transverse View

This eye also demonstrates a split-hyaloid picture along with vitreous hemorrhage, subhyaloid hemorrhage, and partial hemorrhagic posterior vitreous detachment. Interestingly, a break is present along the hyaloid side. Notice that the hyaloid and vitreous cortex look string-like, instead of thread-like, with blood in front of both detachments. In this eye, the aftermovement of the vitreous cortex and hyaloid is undulating.

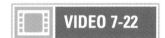

Figure 7-23 Hemorrhagic Vitreoschisis and Hemorrhagic V-Shaped Posterior Vitreous Detachment with Weiss Ring

Horizontal Axial View

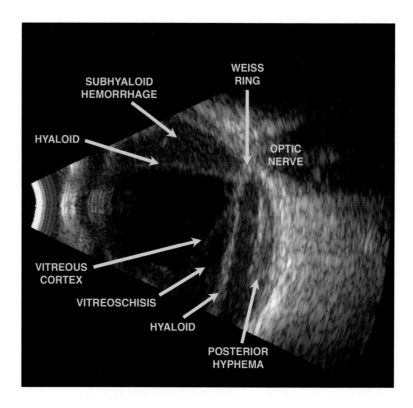

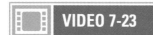

This case depicts a V-shaped hemorrhagic posterior vitreous detachment, with a prominent Weiss ring on the surface of the optic nerve. Note the split-hyaloid picture of the hemorrhagic vitreoschisis at the temporal side (lower half of the scan). Here, blood permeates the schisis and subhyaloid spaces. Posterior hyphema is likewise seen. On dynamic examination, the thread-like vitreous cortex and the atypical string-like hyaloid shake, as subhyaloid blood and the posterior hyphema shift from side to side.

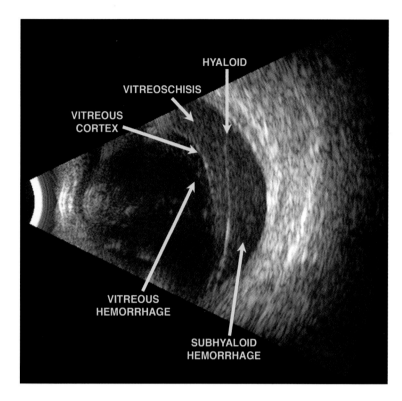

Here is a transverse view of a partial hemorrhagic posterior vitreous
detachment with a split-hyaloid presentation. Here, both the vitreous
cortex and hyaloid appear hair-like. With eye movement, the hyaloid
undulates while the vitreous cortex shakes.

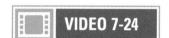

TIP

Vitreoschisis exhibits a split-hyaloid picture in eyes with posterior
vitreous detachments.

Aftermovement of the Retina

8

In contrast to the fine, thread-like appearance of the hyaloid, the retina appears thicker and more string-like when detached from the ocular wall. Retinal detachments (RDs) may occur anywhere in the fundus. The retina has a more varied dynamic ultrasound presentation compared to the rest of the intraocular structures since retinal detachments may be focal or widespread, low-lying or bullous, or open- or closed-funnel in clinical presentation. Most RDs exhibit a shaky form of aftermovement. Some may be jiggly, gradually shifting, or undulating like the vitreous and hyaloid. A few may have no aftermovement at all.

In this chapter, we shall look at focal RD, low-lying RD, retinal breaks or holes, open-funnel RD, closed-funnel RD, traction RD, and retinoschisis.

TIP

When detached, the retina is typically string-like on ultrasound.

Majority: shaky aftermovement

Others: jiggly, shifting, undulating, no aftermovement

FOCAL RETINAL DETACHMENTS

Focal RDs may occur anywhere in the fundus.

Figure 8-1 Serous Focal Retinal Detachment

Horizontal Axial View

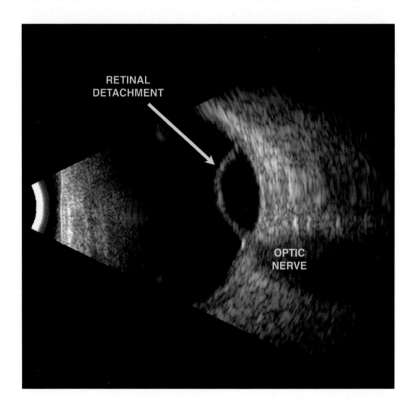

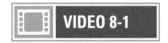

Here, there is a focal, dome-shaped serous retinal detachment immediately nasal to the surface of the optic nerve (upper half of the scan). On dynamic examination, the retina jiggles. A shallower low-lying retinal detachment can also be observed just temporal to the surface of the optic nerve (lower half of the scan).

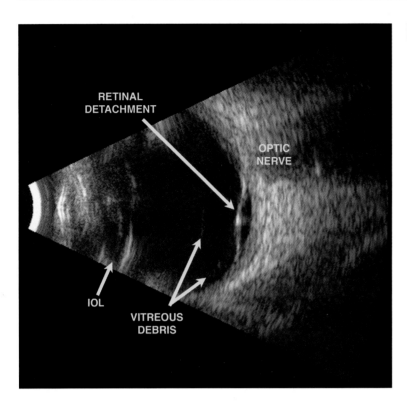

Figure 8-2 Serous Focal Retinal Detachment

Horizontal Axial View

This eye has a focal serous retinal detachment that involves the posterior pole where the macula is located (lower temporal half of the scan). Vitreous debris is likewise present. Here, the retina jiggles.

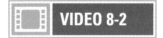

VIDEO 8-2

Figure 8-3 Serous Retinal Detachment, Vitreous Hemorrhage, and Serous Partial Posterior Vitreous Detachment

Vertical Axial View

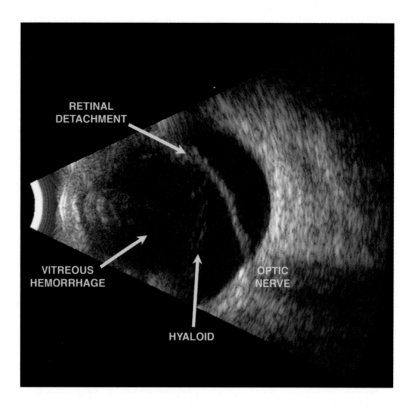

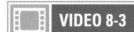

This case depicts vitreous hemorrhage, partial serous posterior vitreous detachment, and a one-sided serous retinal detachment involving the superior fundus (upper half of the scan). In this eye, the retina atypically appears cord-like, resembling the choroid. With eye movement, the retina shakes, while the vitreous and hyaloid undulate. It is important to note that retinal detachments insert along the margins of the optic nerve (the upper margin in this eye), and not away from it as with choroidal detachments (CDs) (see Chapter 9).

TIP

Retinal detachments insert along the margins of the optic nerve, whereas choroidal detachments insert on the sclera away from these margins.

Choroidal tumors may lead to secondary RD. These tumors include retinoblastoma, hemangioma, malignant melanoma, and choroidal granuloma, to name a few.

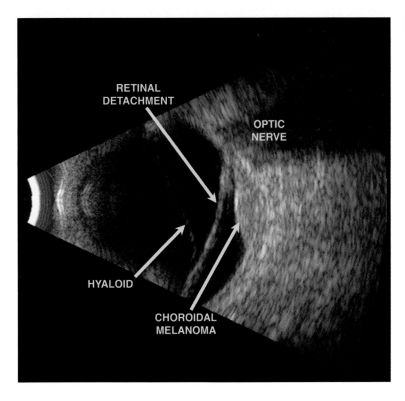

Figure 8-4 Serous Retinal Detachment secondary to Choroidal Melanoma, Serous Complete Posterior Vitreous Detachment

Horizontal Axial View

This eye has a choroidal melanoma at the macular area (temporal lower half of the scan) with overlying retinal detachment. Likewise, a serous type of complete posterior vitreous detachment is also observed. On dynamic examination, the retina shakes while the hyaloid undulates.

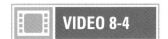

Figure 8-5 Serous Retinal Detachment secondary to Choroidal Melanoma

Transverse View

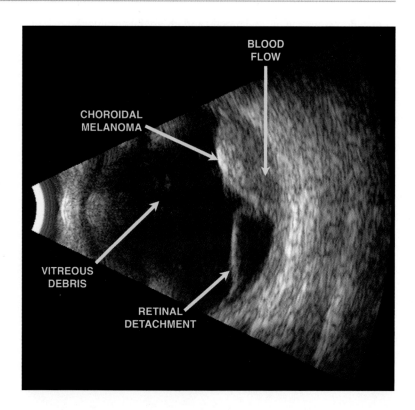

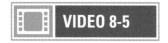

This dome-shaped choroidal melanoma, on the other hand, classically displays a shimmering type of vascularity within the mass. It is also associated with serous retinal detachment. As the eye moves, the retina exhibits a shaky aftermovement.

LOW-LYING RETINAL DETACHMENTS

Like focal RDs, the low-lying variety may be found anywhere in the fundus. Low-lying RDs should always be observed dynamically. They may resemble low-lying PVDs, especially at the periphery where the hyaloid may appear as thick as the retina (see Chapter 7). Additionally, echographic noise (subretinal artifact) may be seen beneath a minimally detached retina, which should not be confused for subretinal hemorrhagic, inflammatory, or tumor cells. Like subhyaloid artifacts, subretinal artifacts are minute, fleeting echobright streaks, as opposed to the more speckled image of cellular particles.

Figure 8-6 Low-Lying Serous Retinal Detachment and Serous Partial Posterior Vitreous Detachment

Peripheral Transverse View

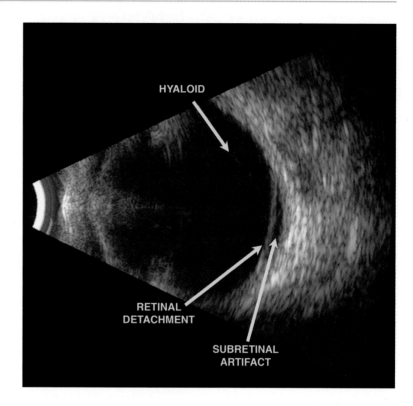

HYALOID

RETINAL DETACHMENT

SUBRETINAL ARTIFACT

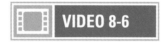

This eye shows a flat, focal serous retinal detachment at the periphery. It is associated with partial serous posterior vitreous detachment where the hyaloid is thread-like. With eye movement, the retina shakes a bit while the hyaloid undulates slightly. Note the presence of a subretinal artifact in this example.

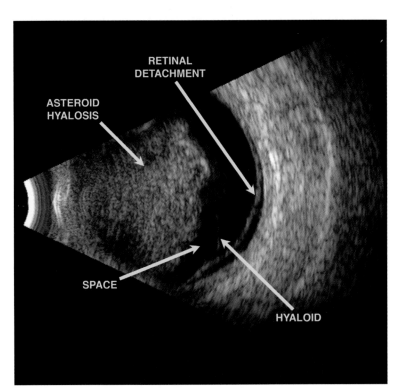

Figure 8-7 Low-Lying Serous Retinal Detachment and Serous Partial Posterior Vitreous Detachment in Asteroid Hyalosis

Peripheral Transverse View

This case demonstrates a low-lying retinal detachment at the periphery and a serous type of partial posterior vitreous detachment. In this eye, the retina is unusually thin. On dynamic examination, the retina shakes, whereas the asteroid-filled vitreous and hyaloid undulate. Note the space that is usually observed between the calcium soaps and the hyaloid (see Fig. 6-1).

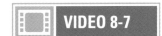

VIDEO 8-7

Figure 8-8 Low-Lying Serous Retinal Detachment and Serous Partial Posterior Vitreous Detachment in Endophthalmitis

Peripheral Transverse View

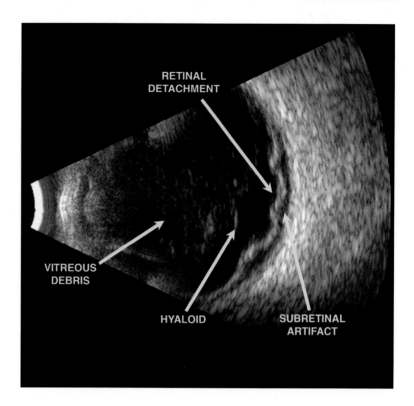

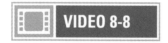

This eye with endophthalmitis presents with partial serous posterior vitreous detachment and low-lying serous retinal detachment. Here, the detached peripheral retina is wavy and appears cord-like in thickness (see Chapter 9). With ocular motion, the retina shakes as both the vitreous and hyaloid undulate.

Retinal Breaks (Holes) at the peripheral fundus may lead to focal, low-lying RDs initially, with a risk of becoming bullous and widespread eventually. Hence, one should be vigilant in screening the retinal periphery for such lesions, particularly in myopic globes, cases with VH from systemic vascular disease, and eyes with a history of trauma.

Longitudinal B-scan views are especially useful for imaging retinal breaks or holes at this location. With this view, retinal breaks are depicted as tiny gaps or openings along the retinal plane, with one or both edges of the break appearing more echobright than the rest of the RD. As a possible cause of rhegmatogenous RD, such findings are easily missed because of their minuscule size.

Figure 8-9 Low-Lying Peripheral Serous Retinal Detachment secondary to Retinal Break, Vitreous Hemorrhage, and Serous Partial Posterior Vitreous Detachment
Peripheral Longitudinal View

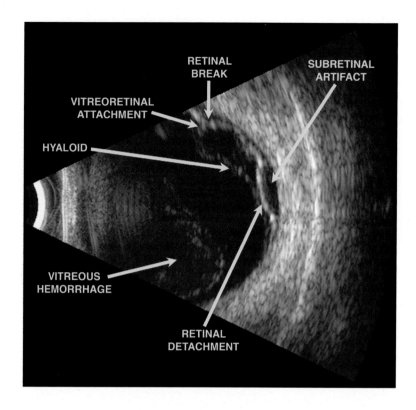

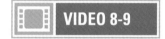

This is an eye with vitreous hemorrhage, partial serous posterior vitreous detachment, and focal low-lying retinal detachment at the periphery. Observe the echobrightness of both edges of the retinal break relative to the elevated retina, as well as the point of vitreoretinal attachment on one side. Subretinal artifact is also present beneath the detachment. On dynamic examination, the retina shakes a bit, while the vitreous and hyaloid undulate.

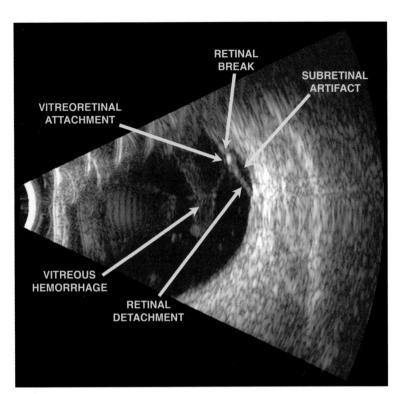

Figure 8-10 Low-Lying Peripheral Serous Retinal Detachment secondary to Retinal Break

Peripheral Longitudinal View

This case is a more peripheral, low-lying retinal detachment. Both edges of the retinal break are more echobright than the rest of the detached retina. In addition, the vitreous hemorrhage appears to have trickled from the retinal break at the point of vitreoretinal attachment. Note that there is minimal movement in this eye, as the focus of examination was on the retinal break.

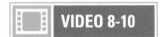

Figure 8-11 Low-Lying Peripheral Retinal Detachment secondary to Retinal Break
Peripheral Longitudinal View

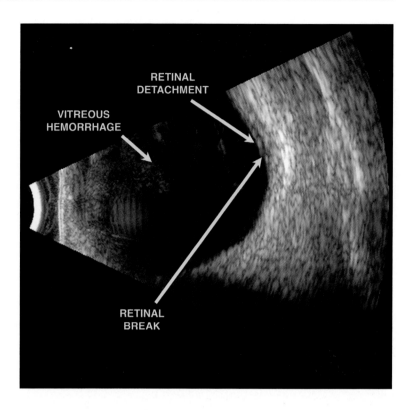

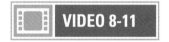

This eye likewise demonstrates a minimally elevated retina at the periphery. Vitreous hemorrhage is also present. Observe the tiny split at the lower end of the retinal detachment, marked by the echobrightness of one edge of the break. Again, the focus of examination was on the retinal break, so ocular tissue movement is scant in this example.

TIP

On longitudinal views, one or both edges of retinal breaks are usually more distinct and echobright compared to the rest of the retinal detachment.

OPEN-FUNNEL RETINAL DETACHMENTS

Open-funnel RDs have a classic V-shaped configuration where the posterior part of the retinal funnel remains open and inserts along the margins of the optic nerve. Open-funnel RDs should be differentiated from V-shaped PVDs, where the base is adherent to the surface of the optic nerve, at times visible as a Weiss ring (see Chapter 7).

Figure 8-12 Serous Open-Funnel Retinal Detachment

Horizontal Axial View

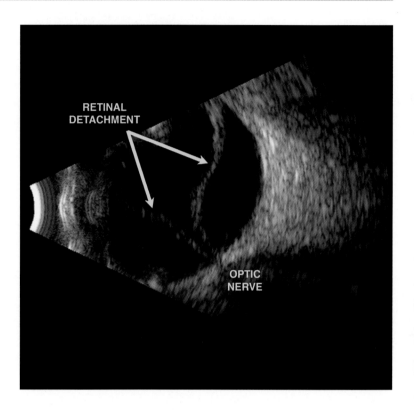

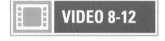

This case exhibits a serous type of V-shaped open-funnel retinal detachment. Note how each side of the string-like, somewhat grainy, retina is inserted along the margins of the optic nerve. On dynamic examination, the retina demonstrates a shaky type of aftermovement.

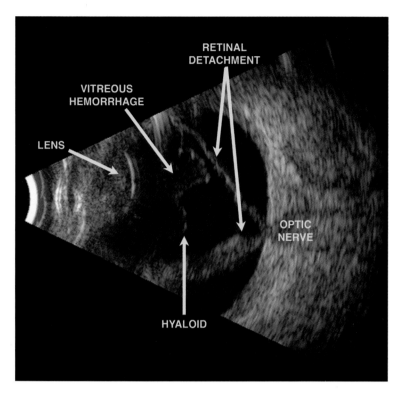

Figure 8-13 Serous Open-Funnel Retinal Detachment, Vitreous Hemorrhage, and Serous Complete Posterior Vitreous Detachment

Horizontal Axial View

This example depicts a V-shaped, serous open-funnel retinal detachment, associated with vitreous hemorrhage and complete serous posterior vitreous detachment. Here, the nasal retina is string-like (top half of the scan), whereas the temporal retina is unusually cord-like and grainy (lower half of the scan) (see Chapter 9). Again, observe the retinal funnel as it inserts along the margins of the optic nerve. With eye movement, the retina shakes, while the vitreous and hyaloid slowly undulate.

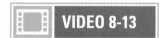

TIP

Open-funnel retinal detachment and V-shaped posterior vitreous detachment have similar ultrasound presentations. However, the base of the former is inserted along the optic nerve margins. In contrast, the base of the latter is attached to the surface of the optic nerve, at times evident as a Weiss ring.

Figure 8-14 Serous Open-Funnel Retinal Detachment, Vitreous, and Subhyaloid Debris with Complete Posterior Vitreous Detachment

Horizontal Axial View

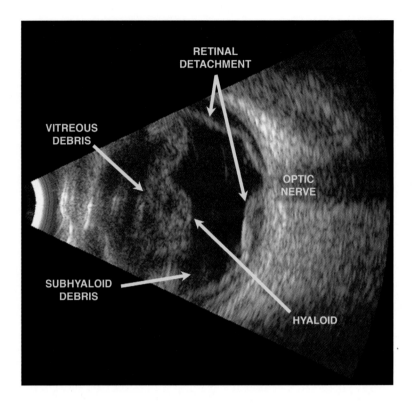

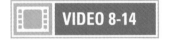

This is an eye with shallow, serous open-funnel retinal detachment, displaying a widened V configuration. Note that the temporal retina appears as thick as the choroid (lower half of the scan), and both sides of the funnel are inserted along the margins of the optic nerve. Other findings are complete posterior vitreous detachment, as well as vitreous and subhyaloid debris. As the eye moves, the retina shakes, while the vitreous and hyaloid undulate.

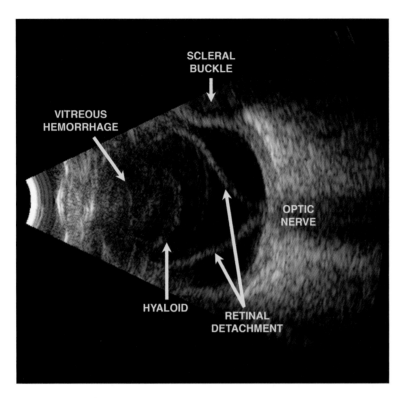

Figure 8-15 Serous Open-Funnel Retinal Detachment, Vitreous Hemorrhage, and Serous Complete Posterior Vitreous Detachment status post Scleral Buckling Procedure

Horizontal Axial View

This case demonstrates a serous open-funnel retinal detachment despite recent scleral buckling surgery. Vitreous hemorrhage and complete posterior vitreous detachment are also present. There is a scleral buckle indentation at the upper equator (top side of the scan). In this eye, observe how the two sides of the string-like retina converge, yet remain separate, as they approach the surface of the optic nerve. On dynamic examination, the retina shakes while the hyaloid undulates.

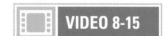

Figure 8-16 Serous Open-Funnel Retinal Detachment, Vitreous Hemorrhage, and Serous Complete Posterior Vitreous Detachment status post Scleral Buckling Procedure

Peripheral Transverse View

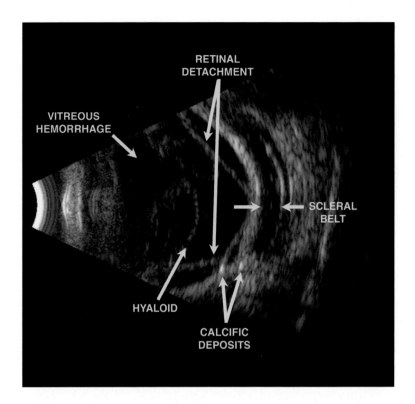

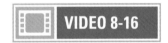

This is a transverse view of the same eye, showing a segment of the scleral belt over the outer surface of the eye. Note the presence of calcific degeneration on the ocular wall, partially shadowing the orbit during eye movement. Again, the retina shakes while the hyaloid undulates.

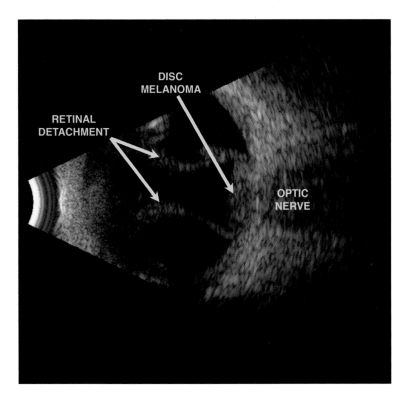

Figure 8-17 Serous Open-Funnel Retinal Detachment secondary to Disc Melanoma
Horizontal Axial View

This case of serous open-funnel retinal detachment is due to a disc melanoma. Here, the contour of the string-like, somewhat grainy, detachment mimics a dome-shaped choroidal detachment, as the girth of the mass has shifted the retina's insertion away from the margins of the optic nerve (see Chapter 9). In this eye, the retina demonstrates a shaky aftermovement. Notice the shimmering type of vascularity within the mass (see Chapter 5).

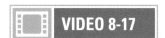

VIDEO 8-17

Figure 8-18 Serous Open-Funnel Retinal
Detachment secondary to Radioactive
Plaque Treatment of Choroidal Melanoma

Transverse View

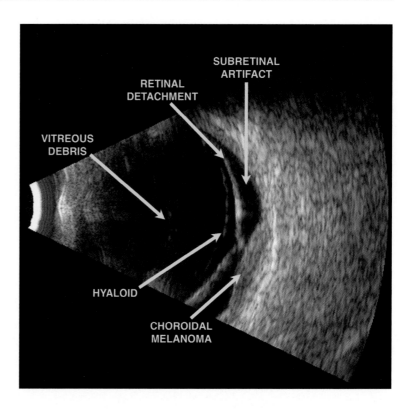

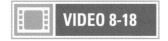

This eye developed a serous open-funnel retinal detachment following radioactive plaque treatment of a choroidal melanoma. In this example, the retina shakes, whereas the vitreous and hyaloid undulate. Observe the presence of subretinal artifact and the absence of a shimmering pulsation within the mass.

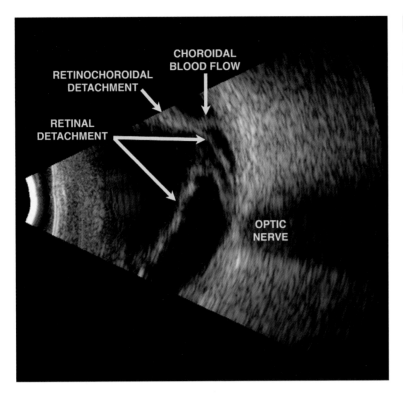

Figure 8-19 Serous Open-Funnel Retinal Detachment and Serous Choroidal Detachment

Vertical Axial View

This eye shows a skewed, serous open-funnel retinal detachment, associated with serous choroidal detachment (see Chapter 9) at the superior equator (top side of the scan). As the eye moves, the more elevated, wavy inferior retina shows minimal shakiness (lower half of the scan), whereas the retinochoroidal detachment remains still. Observe the flow of blood taking place along the choroidal layer (see Chapter 5).

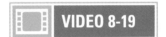

Figure 8-20 Hemorrhagic Open-Funnel Retinal Detachment and Vitreous Hemorrhage

Horizontal Axial View

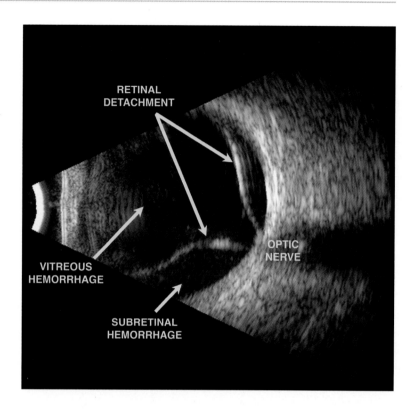

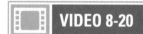

This case depicts a hemorrhagic type of open-funnel retinal detachment, owing to the presence of blood behind the retina. In contrast to the hyaloid that turns echolucent when cellular particles accumulate underneath it, the retina still appears string-like despite pooling of subretinal hemorrhage. Vitreous hemorrhage is likewise seen in this eye. On dynamic examination, the nasal retina shakes (top half of the scan), whereas the vitreous and the temporal retina undulate (lower half of the scan).

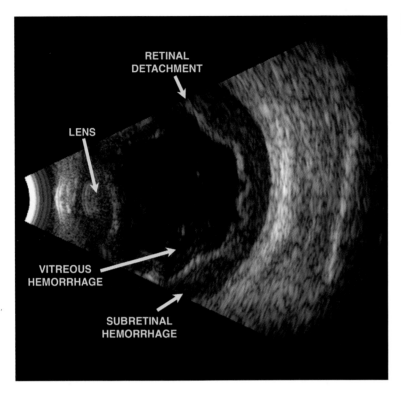

Figure 8-21 Hemorrhagic Open-Funnel Retinal Detachment and Vitreous Hemorrhage
Peripheral Transverse View

This is a peripheral view of the same eye. Here, the wavy looking retina shakes, while the vitreous slowly undulates.

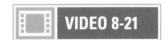

Figure 8-22 Hemorrhagic Open-Funnel
Retinal Detachment and Vitreous
Hemorrhage with Serous Complete Posterior
Vitreous Detachment

Horizontal Axial View

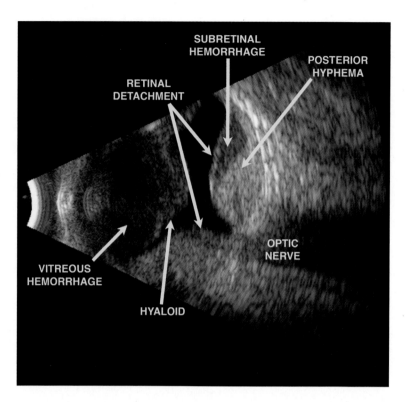

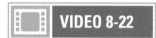

This case of hemorrhagic open-funnel retinal detachment is associated with posterior hyphema within the subretinal space. Observe how the retina still appears string-like despite the subretinal hemorrhage. Vitreous hemorrhage and complete serous posterior vitreous detachment are likewise present. With eye movement, the retina shakes, whereas the vitreous and hyaloid undulate.

In general, the ultrasound picture of ocular tissue detachments becomes modified when hemorrhagic, inflammatory, or tumor cells accumulate in all compartments of the eye. Hence, one should rely less on ultrasound appearance, and more on tissue dynamics, to distinguish the retina from the hyaloid. Observe the following cases.

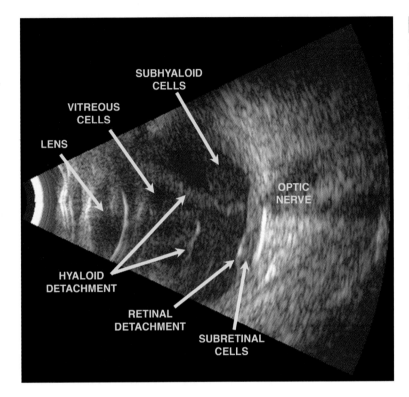

Figure 8-23 Exudative Low-Lying Retinal Detachment and Exudative V-Shaped Posterior Vitreous Detachment in Endophthalmitis
Horizontal Axial View

This eye with endophthalmitis shows an exudative type of V-shaped posterior vitreous detachment and a low-lying exudative retinal detachment involving the posterior pole (lower half of the scan). In this example, dense vitreous and subhyaloid cells modify the appearance and echobrightness of the hyaloid. In turn, dense subhyaloid and subretinal cells modify the image and echobrightness of the retina. As both detachments appear string-like, one has to watch the respective tissue dynamics closely. Here, the retina shakes and the hyaloid undulates.

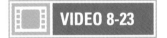

Figure 8-24 Exudative Low-Lying Retinal Detachment and Exudative V-Shaped Posterior Vitreous Detachment in Endophthalmitis

Horizontal Axial View

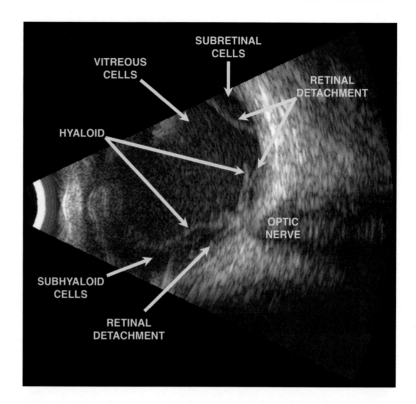

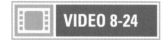

This is another case of endophthalmitis with a V-shaped exudative posterior vitreous detachment and a low-lying exudative retinal detachment. Like the previous example, cells in the vitreous, subhyaloid, and subretinal compartments modify the appearance and echobrightness of the detachments. Upon ocular movement, however, the V-shaped hyaloid detachment undulates a bit, whereas the nasal retinal detachment shakes very slightly (top side of the scan).

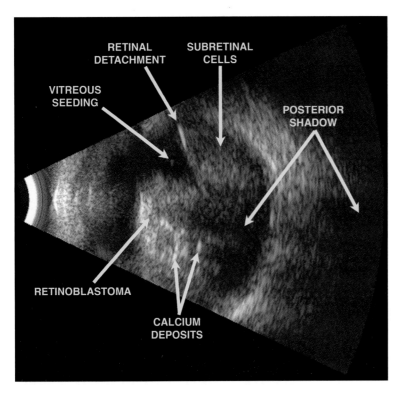

RETINAL
DETACHMENT

SUBRETINAL
CELLS

VITREOUS
SEEDING

POSTERIOR
SHADOW

RETINOBLASTOMA

CALCIUM
DEPOSITS

Figure 8-25 Open-Funnel Retinal Detachment secondary to Endophytic Retinoblastoma

Horizontal Axial View

This case depicts an advanced stage of endophytic retinoblastoma, with a bullous type of secondary open-funnel retinal detachment. In this eye, the retina appears hyaloid-like on account of the density of tumor cells elevating the retina and the posterior shadowing effect of calcium deposits within the mass. During eye movement, the retina displays a shaky aftermovement.

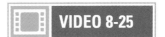 **VIDEO 8-25**

TIP

When cellular particles saturate all compartments of the eye, one should rely more on tissue dynamics, and less on ultrasound appearance, to distinguish the retina from the hyaloid.

Giant Retinal Tears lead to bizarre-looking RDs. In place of the V-shaped profile of open-funnel RDs, a zigzag, coiled, or tortuous configuration is presented.

Figure 8-26 Retinal Detachment secondary to Giant Retinal Tear

Vertical Axial View

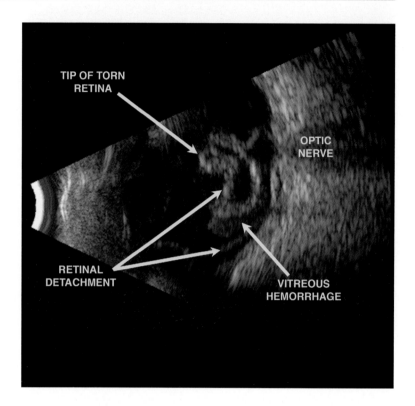

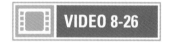

Observe the retinal detachment in this eye. Here, the severed superior retina has coiled in front of the optic nerve, in contrast to the low-lying detachment of the inferior retina. On dynamic examination, the retina shakes, as the vitreous surrounding the coiled retina undulates.

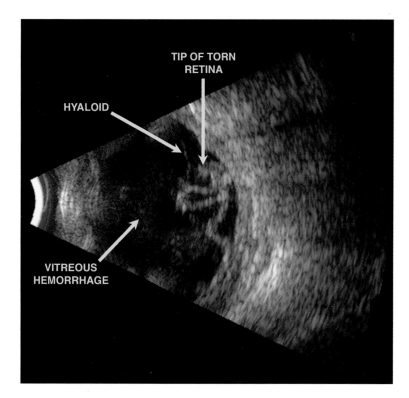

Figure 8-27 Retinal Detachment secondary to Giant Retinal Tear

Longitudinal View

This is a scan of the same eye, where the torn superior retina is displayed in a longitudinal manner (top of the scan is superior peripheral side, bottom is posterior side). Again, the retina shakes, as the vitreous and hyaloid undulate beside it.

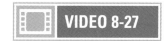

Figure 8-28 Hemorrhagic Retinal Detachment, Serous Choroidal Detachment, and Hemorrhagic Choroidal Effusion secondary to Giant Retinal Tear

Horizontal Axial View

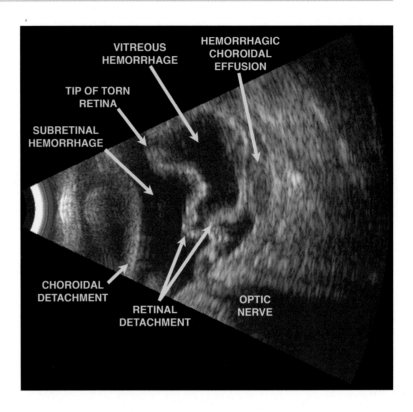

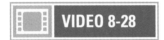

This case presents with a tortuous-looking hemorrhagic retinal detachment, associated with hemorrhagic choroidal effusion nasally (upper half of the scan) and serous choroidal detachment temporally (bottom left side of the scan). Note that one side of the retinal funnel floats freely in the vitreous. Observe the cord-like appearance of the retina (see Chapter 9). With eye movement, the retina shakes while the temporal choroid jiggles.

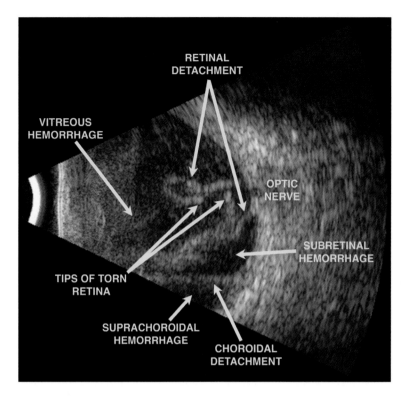

Figure 8-29 Hemorrhagic Retinal Detachment and Hemorrhagic Choroidal Detachment secondary to Giant Retinal Tear

Horizontal Axial View

This eye presents with hemorrhagic retinal detachment and hemorrhagic choroidal detachment owing to the presence of blood in the vitreous (VH), subretinal, and suprachoroidal compartments. On dynamic examination, the bizarrely folded retina shakes, but the choroid on both sides of the equator remains fixed (see Chapter 9). Note the echobright ends of the giant retinal tear, as well as the string-like thickness of the retina and choroid.

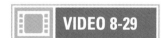

VIDEO 8-29

TIP

Retinal detachments due to giant retinal tears lose their V-shaped profile and exhibit a zigzag, coiled, and tortuous configuration.

Alternatively, to-and-fro movement of eyes with RD may cause subretinal fluid to gradually shift from side to side. This leads to a seesaw-like variation of retinal aftermovement.

Figure 8-30 Serous Focal Retinal Detachment secondary to Choroidal Melanoma

Longitudinal View

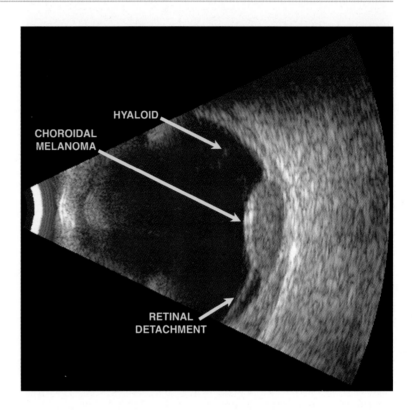

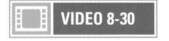

This eye shows a choroidal melanoma at the equator, associated with serous retinal detachment. Here, the retina is typically string-like. Observe the shifting type of retinal aftermovement, as the vitreous and hyaloid undulate.

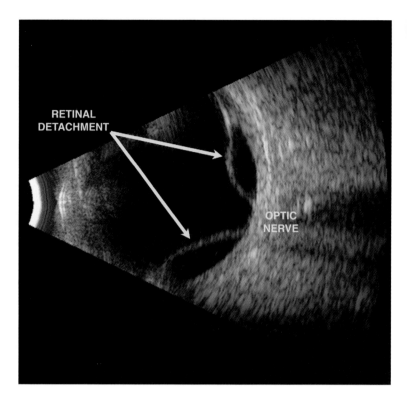

Figure 8-31 Serous Open-Funnel Retinal Detachment

Horizontal Axial View

This case shows an open-funnel type of serous retinal detachment. Again, the retina is characteristically string-like. On dynamic examination, it also displays a shifting type of aftermovement.

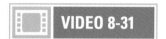

Figure 8-32   Serous Retinal Detachment, Vitreous Hemorrhage, and Serous Complete Posterior Vitreous Detachment

Transverse View

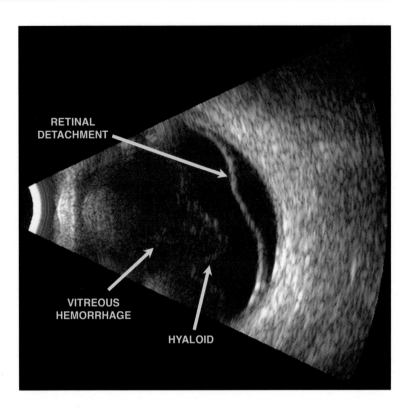

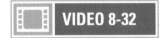

This is a peripheral scan of a case depicting vitreous hemorrhage, complete serous posterior vitreous detachment, and serous retinal detachment. With eye movement, the string-like retina shifts, while the vitreous and thread-like hyaloid undulate.

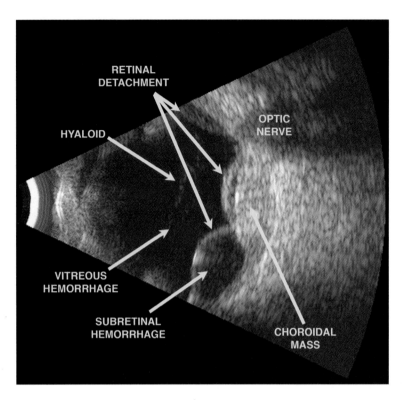

Figure 8-33 Hemorrhagic Open-Funnel Retinal Detachment secondary to Choroidal Mass, Serous Partial Posterior Vitreous Detachment

Horizontal Axial View

This eye has partial serous posterior vitreous detachment as well as hemorrhagic open-funnel retinal detachment secondary to a choroidal mass at the macula (lower half of the scan). Here, the string-like retina shifts, while the vitreous and the thread-like hyaloid undulate with eye movement.

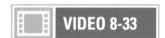

Figure 8-34 Hemorrhagic Open-Funnel Retinal Detachment secondary to Collar-Button Choroidal Melanoma

Horizontal Para-axial View

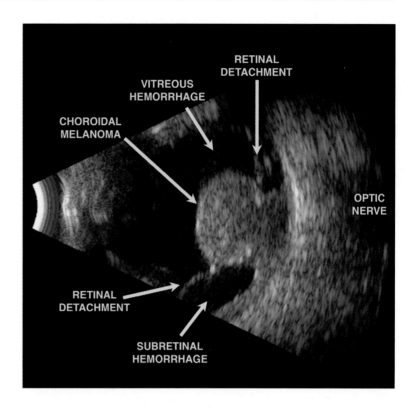

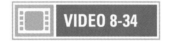

This case exhibits a mushroom-shaped choroidal melanoma with secondary hemorrhagic, open-funnel retinal detachment. In the presence of subretinal blood, the retina has become indiscernible. On dynamic examination, retinal aftermovement is notably shifting.

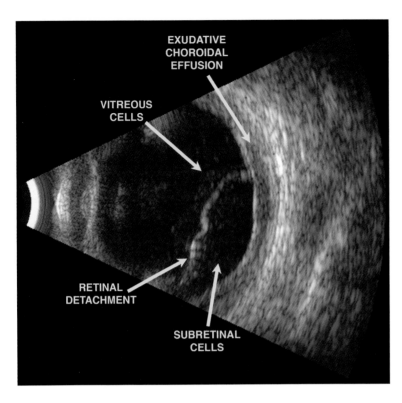

EXUDATIVE
CHOROIDAL
EFFUSION

VITREOUS
CELLS

RETINAL
DETACHMENT

SUBRETINAL
CELLS

Figure 8-35 Exudative Retinal Detachment and Exudative Choroidal Effusion in Endophthalmitis

Transverse View

This is an eye with endophthalmitis. Note that the exudative retinal detachment is associated with exudative choroidal effusion. Again, the string-like retina shifts, as the vitreous and subretinal debris swirl on dynamic examination.

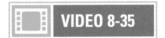

VIDEO 8-35

Figure 8-36 Exudative Open-Funnel Retinal Detachment and Exudative Choroidal Effusion in Endophthalmitis

Horizontal Axial View

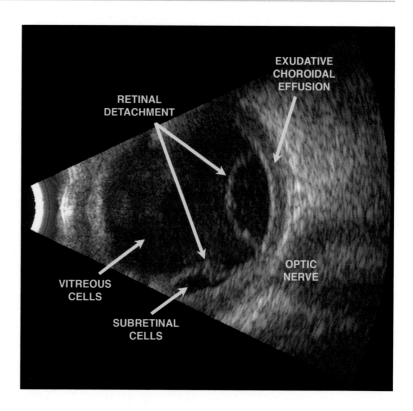

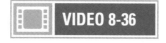

This case of open-funnel exudative retinal detachment from endophthalmitis displays two forms of aftermovement: the temporal retina with the frayed end shakes (lower half of the scan), whereas the nasal retina shifts (upper half of the scan). In this example, the retina appears string-like but grainy, because of the presence of cells in both the vitreous and subretinal compartments. Note the associated exudative choroidal effusion in this eye.

Interestingly, the retina may exhibit an undulating motion similar to the aftermovement of the hyaloid. This variant of retinal aftermovement may be observed in longstanding posterior uveitis, endophthalmitis, or eyes that have had severe trauma in the past.

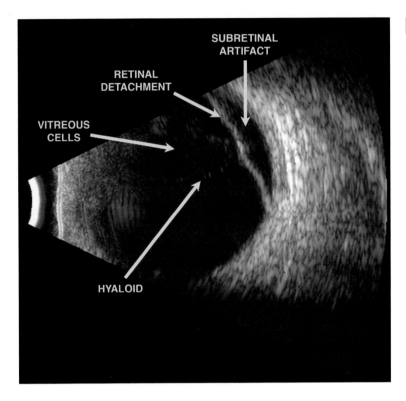

Figure 8-37 Serous Focal Retinal Detachment and Serous Partial Posterior Vitreous Detachment in Chronic Posterior Uveitis

Longitudinal View

This case is from an eye with chronic posterior uveitis. It shows a partial serous posterior vitreous detachment and a focal serous retinal detachment at the fundus periphery. Note the subretinal artifact usually observed in low-lying detachments. With motion, the atypically cord-like retina displays an unusual wiggly undulation, while the thread-like hyaloid undulates beside it.

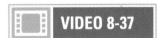

VIDEO 8-37

Figure 8-38 Serous Open-Funnel Retinal Detachment and V-Shaped Posterior Vitreous Detachment in Chronic Posterior Uveitis

Horizontal Axial View

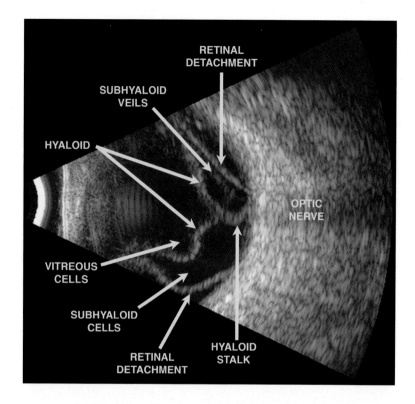

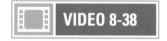

This eye with long-standing posterior uveitis presents with a wide, open-funnel serous retinal detachment as well as a V-shaped posterior vitreous detachment. Note that the hyaloid is attached directly on the surface of the optic nerve, while the nasal retina is inserted along the optic nerve margin (upper half of the scan). In this eye, both the hyaloid and the retina appear unusually cord-like (see Chapter 9). On dynamic examination, the retina undulates along with the vitreous, hyaloid, and subhyaloid cells and veils.

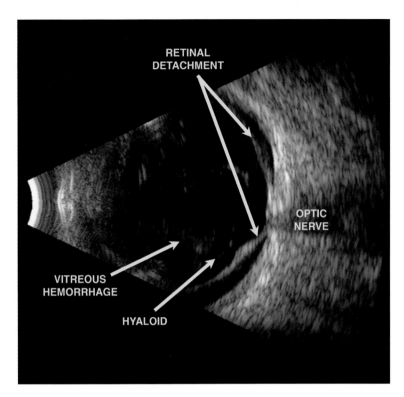

RETINAL
DETACHMENT

OPTIC
NERVE

VITREOUS
HEMORRHAGE

HYALOID

Figure 8-39 Serous Open-Funnel Retinal Detachment and Serous Complete Posterior Vitreous Detachment status post Old Trauma

Horizontal Axial View

This eye sustained trauma in the past. Significant findings include vitreous hemorrhage, complete serous posterior vitreous detachment, and wide, open-funnel serous retinal detachment. In this example, the string-like retina appears to taper toward the sides. On dynamic examination, both the retina and the thread-like hyaloid exhibit an undulating type of aftermovement.

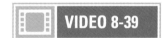

VIDEO 8-39

Figure 8-40 Serous Retinal Detachment secondary to Choroidal Granuloma, Vitreous Debris, and Serous Partial Posterior Vitreous Detachment

Peripheral Longitudinal View

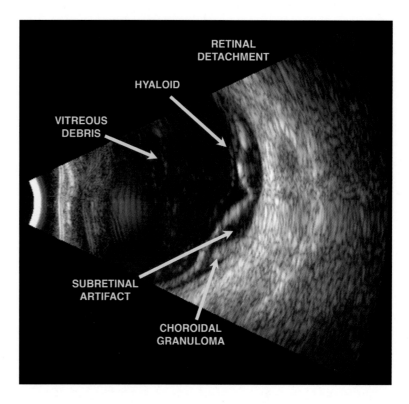

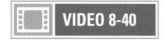

This scan depicts a pedunculated choroidal granuloma, with secondary serous retinal detachment. Overlying vitreous debris and partial serous posterior vitreous detachment are likewise present. Here, the retina appears wavy and atypically cord-like (see Chapter 9). As the eye moves, the retina undulates a bit relative to the undulation of the thread-like hyaloid. Observe the subretinal artifact during eye movement.

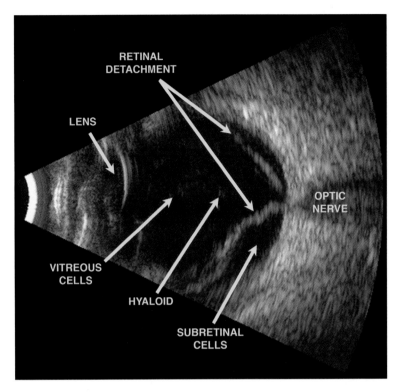

Figure 8-41 Exudative Open-Funnel Retinal Detachment and Serous Partial Posterior Vitreous Detachment in Endophthalmitis

Horizontal Axial View

This eye with chronic endophthalmitis displays partial serous posterior vitreous detachment and an open-funnel type of exudative retinal detachment with fine cells in the subretinal compartment. Here, the vitreous is filled with cellular debris, and the retina is unusually cord-like, grainy and frayed. Observe the retina as it undulates along with the thread-like hyaloid.

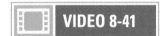 **VIDEO 8-41**

Figure 8-42 Hemorrhagic Retinal Detachment, Vitreous Hemorrhage, and Serous Complete Posterior Vitreous Detachment status post Old Trauma

Peripheral Transverse View

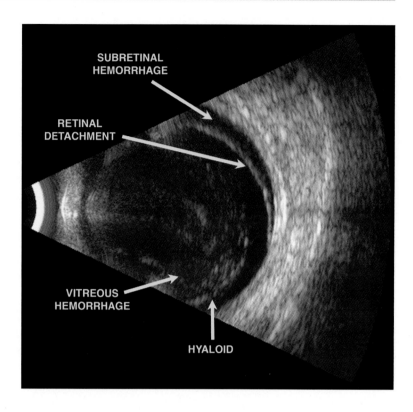

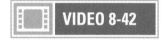

This peripheral scan is taken from an eye that had severe trauma in the past. Significant findings include vitreous hemorrhage, complete serous posterior vitreous detachment, and hemorrhagic retinal detachment. Upon eye movement, the frayed, string-like retina undulates slowly along with the vitreous and thread-like hyaloid.

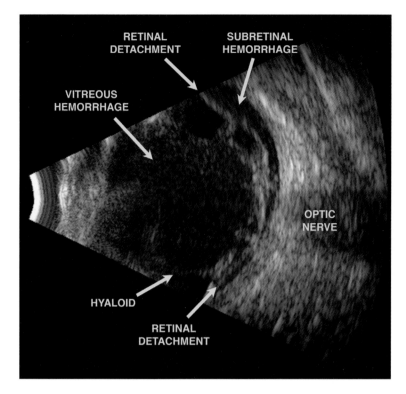

Figure 8-43 Hemorrhagic Open-Funnel Retinal Detachment, Vitreous Hemorrhage, and Serous Partial Posterior Vitreous Detachment in Ruptured Globe
Horizontal Axial View

This eye sustained recent traumatic globe rupture. It presents with a low-lying, open-funnel hemorrhagic retinal detachment. In this example, vitreous hemorrhage and partial serous posterior vitreous detachment are also present. On dynamic examination, both the thread-like hyaloid and the string-like retina exhibit a restricted type of undulation.

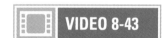

VIDEO 8-43

Figure 8-44 Hemorrhagic Open-Funnel Retinal Detachment, Vitreous Hemorrhage, and Serous Partial Posterior Vitreous Detachment in Ruptured Globe

Peripheral Transverse View

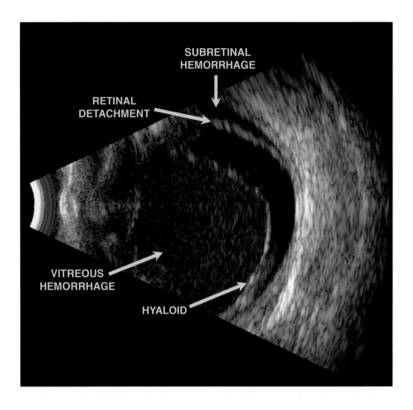

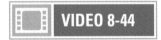

This is a transverse view of the same eye. The undulation of the hyaloid and the retina is also limited. Note that the atypically string-like hyaloid tapers and becomes segmented halfway up, whereas the retina appears uniformly string-like from end to end. These echographic differences help distinguish the hyaloid from the retina.

TIP

Retinal undulation may be observed in eyes with long-standing intraocular inflammation or a past history of severe trauma.

CLOSED-FUNNEL RETINAL DETACHMENTS

Closed-funnel RDs may exhibit a triangular-, cocoon-, or T-shaped configuration, with the posterior end of the funnel fused or closed as it approaches the optic disc. These detachments may be serous, hemorrhagic, or exudative in nature. Compared to the serous type, the hemorrhagic or exudative variety is more daunting to diagnose because of the masking effect of cellular debris surrounding the retinal funnel. One may have to vary the orientation of the probe, say from horizontal axial to vertical axial position, to detect its presence in the eye.

Most closed-funnel RDs are chronic, as evidenced by the onset of cystic and/or calcific degeneration. Moreover, most do not exhibit any retinal aftermovement. Closed-funnel RDs should be differentiated from V-shaped PVDs that exhibit thick hyaloid stalks adherent to the surface of the optic nerve (see Chapter 7 and Fig. 8-63).

Figure 8-45 Serous Triangular Retinal Detachment in Phthisis Bulbi

Horizontal Axial View

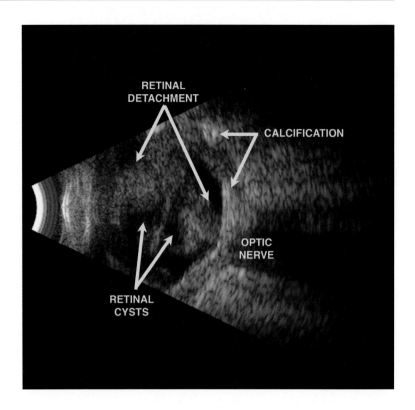

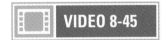

This case depicts a closed-funnel serous retinal detachment in a phthisical eye. Here, the detachment has a triangular, bunch-of-grapes configuration arising from cystic retinal degeneration. The grainy appearance of the detachment, thickened and calcified ocular wall, and shrunken globe are findings consistent with phthisis bulbi. No retinal aftermovement is observed in this eye.

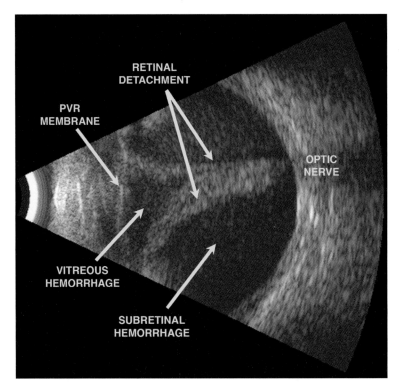

Figure 8-46 Hemorrhagic Triangular Retinal Detachment and Vitreous Hemorrhage
Horizontal Axial View

This is another eye demonstrating a triangular hemorrhagic retinal detachment. With dense vitreous hemorrhage and subretinal hemorrhage, the retina appears grainy and cord-like (see Chapter 9). Note that the retinal funnel has become narrow from proliferative vitreoretinopathy (PVR). On dynamic examination, the retina shakes vigorously.

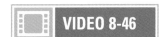

VIDEO 8-46

Figure 8-47 Hemorrhagic Triangular Retinal Detachment

Horizontal Axial View

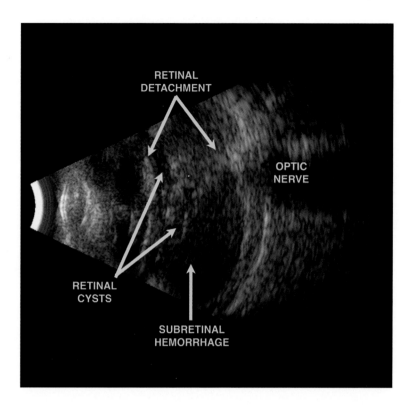

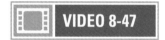

The closed-funnel hemorrhagic retinal detachment in this example is indiscernible because of dense cellular debris. With eye movement, the detachment can be outlined as a triangular, bunch-of-grapes configuration, with retinal cysts present anteriorly. Here, subretinal blood shifts around, but the retina shows no aftermovement. Note that this scan was obtained with the probe in a horizontal position.

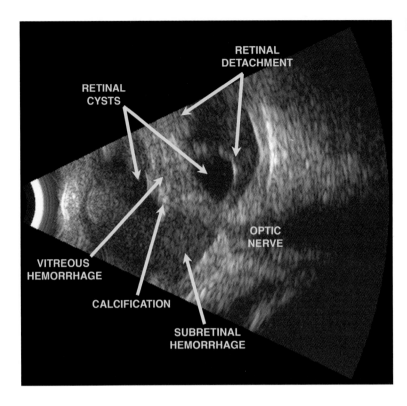

RETINAL
DETACHMENT

RETINAL
CYSTS

OPTIC
NERVE

VITREOUS
HEMORRHAGE

CALCIFICATION

SUBRETINAL
HEMORRHAGE

Figure 8-48 Hemorrhagic Triangular Retinal Detachment

Vertical Axial View

This is a scan of the same eye obtained with the probe in a vertical position. This time, the outline of the hemorrhagic retinal detachment and its cysts are more apparent, with the retina appearing grainy from calcific degeneration. Again, the retina remains fixed.

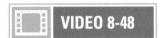

VIDEO 8-48

Figure 8-49 Hemorrhagic Triangular Retinal Detachment

Horizontal Axial View

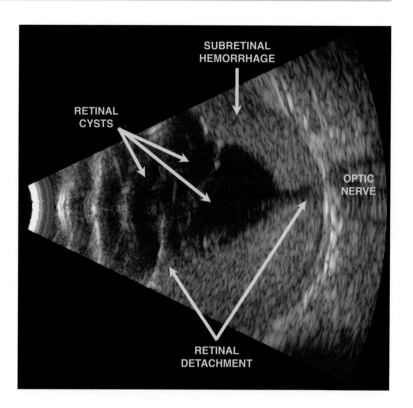

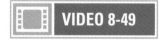

This case of closed-funnel hemorrhagic retinal detachment displays large, serous retinal cysts. Again, the retina shows a triangular, bunch-of-grapes configuration. On dynamic examination, the retina shakes, while blood shifts back and forth outside the funnel.

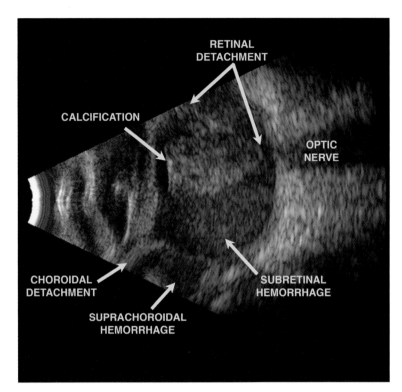

Figure 8-50 Hemorrhagic Triangular Retinal Detachment and Hemorrhagic Choroidal Detachment
Horizontal Axial View

This eye also has a triangular hemorrhagic retinal detachment. Here, the associated findings are calcific degeneration, as well as hemorrhagic choroidal detachments at the nasal and temporal equator (top and bottom sides of the scan, respectively). With eye movement, the retinal calcifications cast shadows posteriorly, while blood swirls from side to side outside the funnel and beneath the choroid. However, both retinal and choroidal aftermovements are absent.

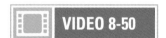 **VIDEO 8-50**

TIP

A triangular, bunch-of-grapes configuration in a closed-funnel retinal detachment is mainly a result of cystic retinal degeneration.

Figure 8-51 Hemorrhagic Cocoon-Shaped
Retinal Detachment

Horizontal Axial View

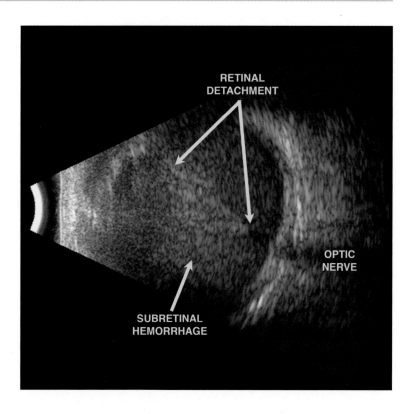

RETINAL
DETACHMENT

OPTIC
NERVE

SUBRETINAL
HEMORRHAGE

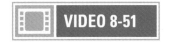

In this case, the amount of subretinal blood is so dense that the outline of a cocoon-shaped, closed-funnel hemorrhagic retinal detachment is barely perceptible. On dynamic examination, subretinal blood shifts to and fro, but the retina remains fixed.

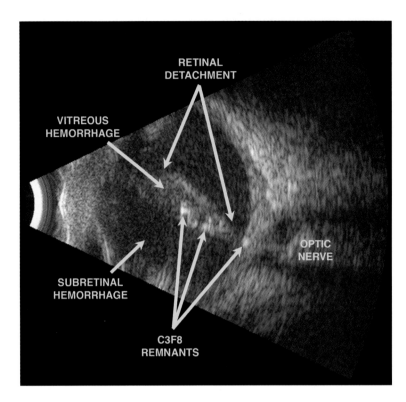

Figure 8-52 Hemorrhagic Cocoon-Shaped Retinal Detachment with C3F8 Remnants
Horizontal Axial View

Here is an indistinct, cocoon-shaped hemorrhagic retinal detachment, with C3F8 gas remaining from a surgical procedure in the past. C3F8 gas is known to adhere to the retina, and it casts multiple echobright signals posteriorly. In this eye, the retina appears grainy with the cellular debris. As it moves, vitreous and subretinal blood is set in motion, but no retinal aftermovement is observed.

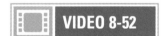

Figure 8-53 Serous T-Shaped Retinal Detachment

Horizontal Axial View

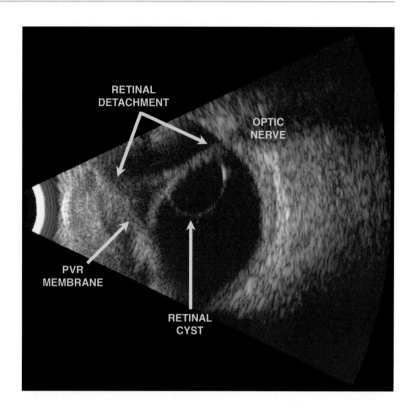

RETINAL DETACHMENT

OPTIC NERVE

PVR MEMBRANE

RETINAL CYST

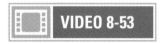

This case is a T-shaped, closed-funnel serous retinal detachment. Here, a huge retinal cyst bulges temporally (lower side of the scan). T-shaped retinal detachments usually result from proliferative vitreoretinopathy (PVR). On dynamic examination, the anterior retinal funnel shakes.

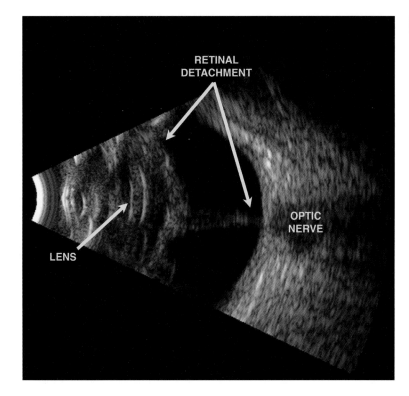

Figure 8-54 Serous T-Shaped Retinal Detachment

Horizontal Axial View

This eye also presents a T-shaped serous retinal detachment. In this example, the retina is echolucent. With eye movement, the anterior end of the funnel is noted to shake.

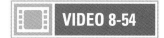

Figure 8-55 Serous T-Shaped Retinal Detachment

Horizontal Axial View

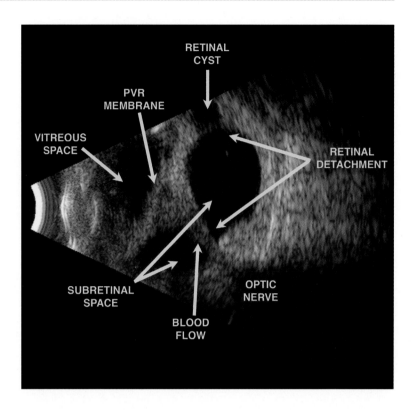

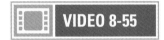

This case exhibits a more solid-looking, T-shaped serous retinal detachment from proliferative vitreoretinopathy. Here, the retina is grossly thickened and associated with a retinal cyst anteriorly (top side of the scan). Choroidal thickening is likewise present. As the eye moves, retinal blood flow can be observed along the base of the detachment, but no retinal aftermovement can be observed.

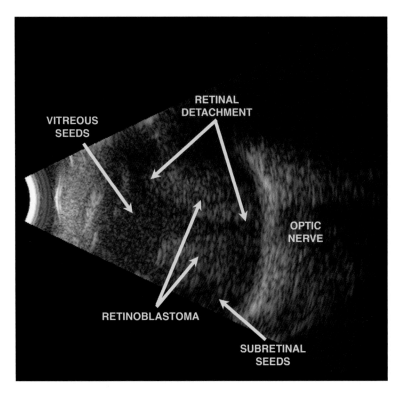

Figure 8-56 T-Shaped Retinal Detachment secondary to Exophytic Retinoblastoma
Horizontal Axial View

This case depicts a T-shaped retinal detachment secondary to exophytic retinoblastoma. In this eye, only a silhouette of the closed-funnel retinal detachment is visible due to the size of the mass surrounding the funnel. On dynamic examination, vitreous, and subretinal seeds shift slightly, but the retina shows no aftermovement.

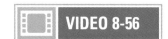

Figure 8-57 Exudative T-Shaped Retinal Detachment secondary to Coats Disease
Horizontal Axial View

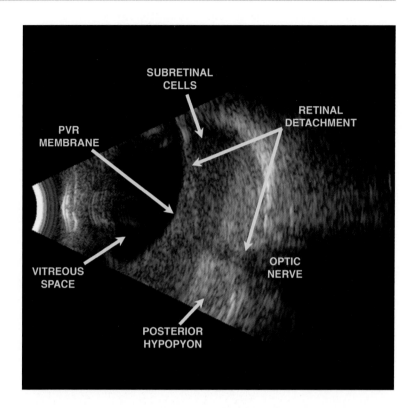

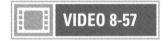

In Coats disease, a profusion of subretinal exudates eventually leads to retinal detachment. Here, the T-shaped exudative retinal detachment is rendered echolucent by dense cellular debris surrounding the funnel. Its silhouette becomes evident only upon eye movement. Observe the subretinal cells and posterior hypopyon shifting from side to side. However, no retinal aftermovement can be seen.

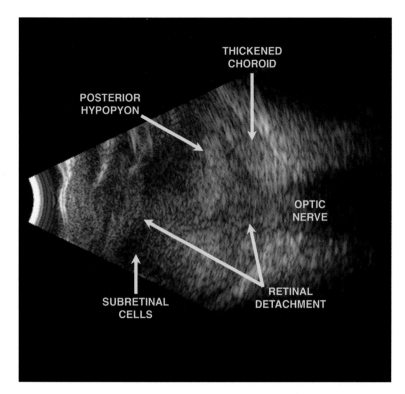

POSTERIOR
HYPOPYON

THICKENED
CHOROID

OPTIC
NERVE

SUBRETINAL
CELLS

RETINAL
DETACHMENT

Figure 8-58 Exudative T-Shaped Retinal Detachment in Chronic Posterior Uveitis
Horizontal Axial View

This eye exhibits a T-shaped exudative retinal detachment from chronic posterior uveitis. Here, dense posterior hypopyon and choroidal thickening are also present. Upon eye movement, a grainy outline of the closed-funnel retinal detachment is uncovered. Apart from the to-and-fro motion of the posterior hypopyon and subretinal cells, no retinal aftermovement can be observed.

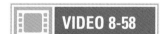

VIDEO 8-58

Figure 8-59 Hemorrhagic T-Shaped Retinal Detachment with Serous Retinal Cyst

Horizontal Axial View

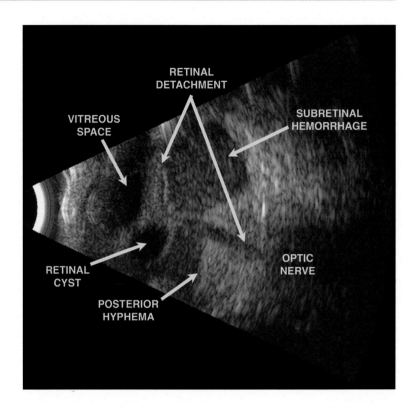

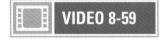

This case shows a proliferative vitreoretinopathy-induced, T-shaped hemorrhagic retinal detachment, with a serous retinal cyst temporally (lower side of the scan). In this eye, the retina is barely discernible on account of blood surrounding the funnel. Here, the posterior hyphema and subretinal blood shift with eye movement, but the retina remains stiff.

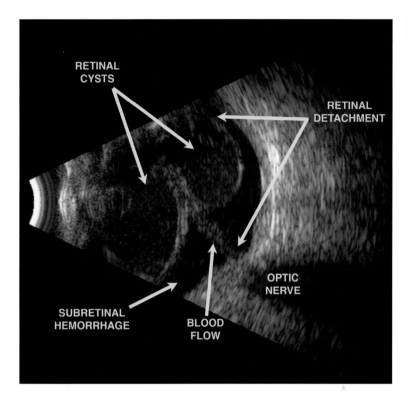

Figure 8-60 Hemorrhagic T-Shaped Retinal Detachment with Hemorrhagic Retinal Cysts
Horizontal Axial View

Likewise, this eye presents a T-shaped hemorrhagic retinal detachment resulting from proliferative vitreoretinopathy. Here, two huge hemorrhagic retinal cysts flank the sides of the funnel. On dynamic examination, the retina demonstrates a jiggly form of aftermovement. Notice the motion of blood within the cysts and subretinal space, as well as the rapid flow of blood along the apposed retina.

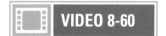

Figure 8-61 Hemorrhagic T-Shaped Retinal Detachment with Posterior Lens Dislocation

Horizontal Axial View

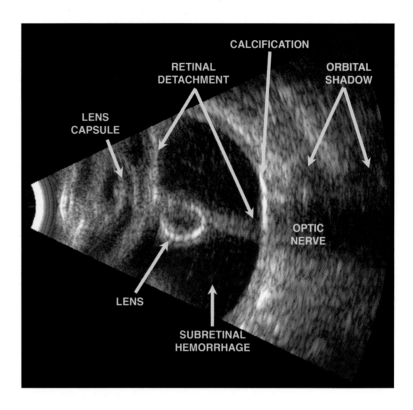

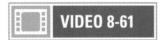

Interestingly, this eye exhibits a dislocated cataractous lens, trapped within a T-shaped hemorrhagic retinal detachment. Again, the retina appears grainy through the cellular debris. With eye movement, the anterior end of the funnel jiggles a bit, while the empty lens capsule anterior to the funnel shifts from side to side. Moreover, observe the patch of calcific degeneration at the nasal part of the globe that shadows the orbit (posterior part of the scan).

TIP

In eyes with dense cellular debris, it may be necessary to vary the position of the probe to unmask the presence of a closed-funnel retinal detachment.

TRACTION RETINAL DETACHMENTS

Traction retinal detachments (TRDs) generally have no aftermovement. Traction usually arises from vitreous bands or preretinal membranes that contract and pull the retina to varying degrees of elevation. Foremost among the possible causes of TRD is diabetic retinopathy, where traction may assume a tent-like or tabletop configuration.

Figure 8-62 Tent-Like Traction Retinal Detachment and Hemorrhagic V-Shaped Posterior Vitreous Detachment with Hemorrhagic Vitreoschisis

Horizontal Axial View

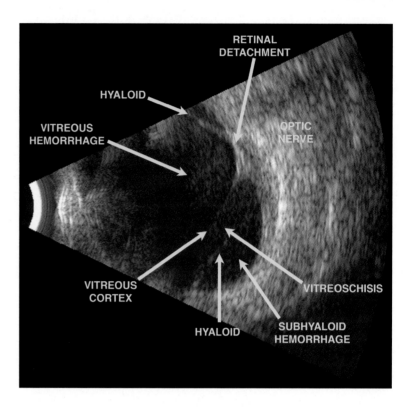

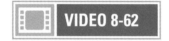

This eye shows a hemorrhagic V-shaped posterior vitreous detachment associated with a tent-like retinal detachment in the vicinity of the optic nerve. The nasal hyaloid appears string-like from the effect of blood in the vitreous and subhyaloid compartments (upper side of the scan). The temporal hyaloid shows a split-hyaloid picture (see Chapter 7), with the hyaloid retaining its thread-like appearance (lower half of the scan). As the eye moves, the hyaloid shakes, the walls of the temporal vitreoschisis undulate, but the elevated retina remains rigid.

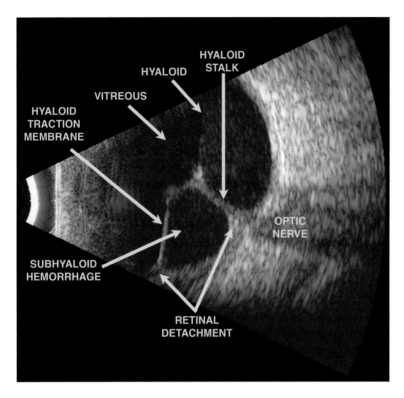

Figure 8-63 Tent-Like Peripapillary and Macular Traction Retinal Detachment
Horizontal Axial View

This case resembles a T-shaped closed funnel retinal detachment. In this example, a thick hyaloid stalk lifts the retina in the vicinity of the optic nerve. A smaller tent-like elevation is likewise present at the temporal macula (bottom of the scan). Observe that the anterior part of the hyaloid extending nasally from the center of the vitreous cavity has become indiscernible in the presence of dense subhyaloid hemorrhage (upper half of the scan). Aside from the to-and-fro motion of subhyaloid blood, no retinal nor hyaloid aftermovement can be seen in this eye with tent-like peripapillary and macular traction retinal detachments.

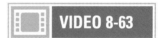

VIDEO 8-63

Figure 8-64 Tent-Like Traction Retinal Detachment secondary to Preretinal Membrane, Serous V-Shaped Posterior Vitreous Detachment

Horizontal Axial View

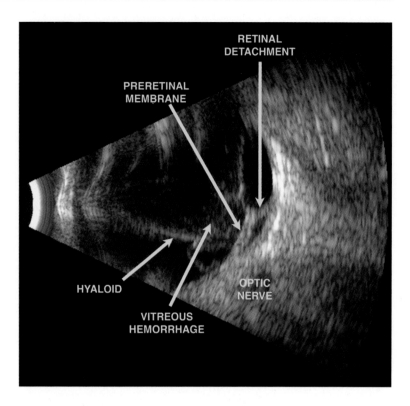

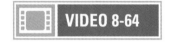

This eye shows a V-shaped serous posterior vitreous detachment, with a tent-like traction retinal detachment just nasal to the surface of the optic nerve. Note the presence of a preretinal membrane over the lower half of the elevated retina close to the optic nerve. On dynamic examination, the vitreous hemorrhage and the hyaloid undulate, but the tented retina stays fixed.

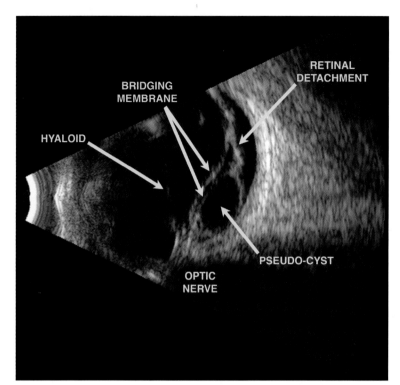

Figure 8-65 Tent-Like Serous Traction Retinal Detachment with Pseudocyst secondary to Bridging Membrane

Longitudinal Temporal View

This is a longitudinal view of an eye, where the temporal retina demonstrates a tent-like, serous detachment of the macula. Here, the preretinal bridging membrane and the tented retina are in a ring-like formation that could be misinterpreted to be a retinal cyst instead of a pseudocyst. As with most cases of traction retinal detachment, retinal aftermovement is absent.

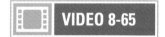

Figure 8-66 Tent-Like Hemorrhagic Traction Retinal Detachment with Pseudocyst secondary to Bridging Membrane, Hemorrhagic V-Shaped Posterior Vitreous Detachment

Horizontal Para-axial View

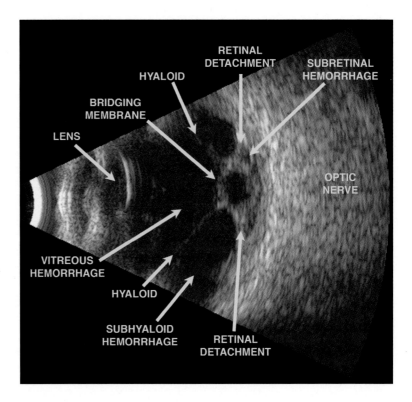

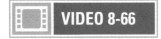
VIDEO 8-66

This case exhibits a hemorrhagic V-shaped posterior vitreous detachment. In this eye, there are two tent-like hemorrhagic traction retinal detachments that are bridged by a membrane in the vicinity of the optic nerve. Consequently, a ring-like structure or pseudocyst is formed that could be mistaken for a vitreous cyst (see Fig. 6-6). Both vitreous hemorrhage and subhyaloid hemorrhage are likewise present. On dynamic examination, the preretinal bridging membrane unfolds and partly undulates, whereas the hyaloid shakes. However, the thickened retina shows no aftermovement.

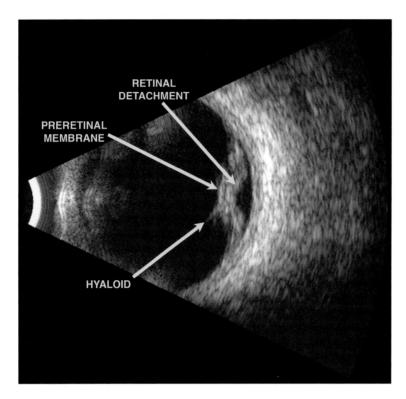

Figure 8-67 Tabletop Serous Traction Retinal Detachment secondary to Preretinal Membrane

Transverse View

This eye depicts serous traction retinal detachment, with the retina forming a tabletop configuration. Here, the elevated retina appears very thick as a result of a thickened preretinal membrane. Note that the hyaloid elevating it is indiscernible. Again, no retinal aftermovement can be observed in this eye.

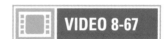

Figure 8-68 Tabletop Hemorrhagic Traction Retinal Detachment secondary to Preretinal Membrane

Transverse View

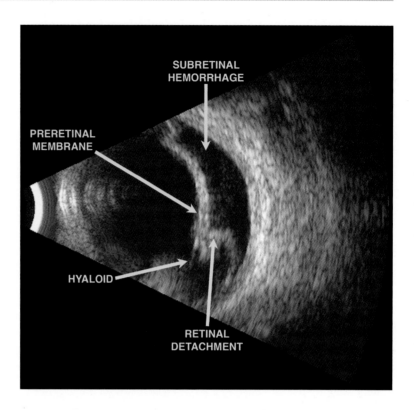

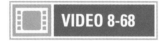

This example exhibits a much wider, tabletop form of hemorrhagic traction retinal detachment, with only part of the hyaloid visible to the eye. Observe the thickened detachment due to the preretinal membrane. In this eye, subretinal hemorrhage is likewise noted. Again, the retina remains fixed during eye movement.

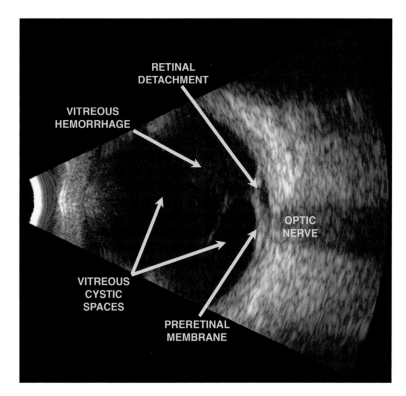

Figure 8-69 Focal Traction Retinal Detachment secondary to Preretinal Membrane

Horizontal Axial View

This case of focal traction retinal detachment shows a thick membrane on the surface of the optic nerve. Here, the nasal retina is elevated in the absence of traction from the hyaloid (upper half of the scan). Vitreous hemorrhage is also present. On dynamic examination, vitreous undulation is observed, but no retinal aftermovement is appreciated. Note the cystic spaces in the vitreous and compare them with true vitreous cysts (see Figs. 6-6 and 7-13).

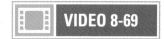

Figure 8-70 Hemorrhagic Open-Funnel Traction Retinal Detachment secondary to Preretinal Membrane, Serous V-Shaped Posterior Vitreous Detachment

Horizontal Axial View

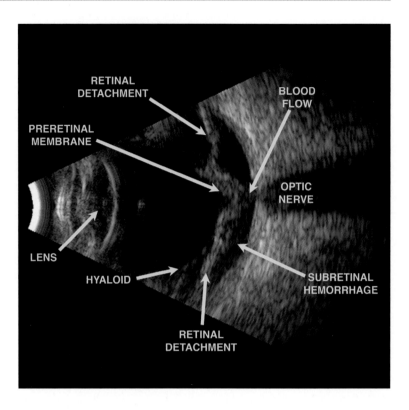

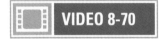

This eye demonstrates an open-funnel type of hemorrhagic traction retinal detachment. There is a thick preretinal membrane on the surface of the optic nerve and peripapillary retina, which appears to have elevated the retina on both sides. With eye movement, the temporal retina and the wide, V-shaped serous posterior vitreous detachment shake minimally (lower half of the scan). Observe the flow of blood along the nasal retina close to the disc.

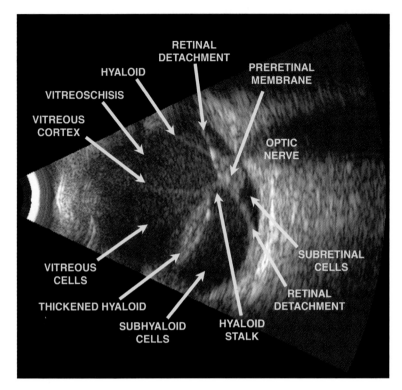

Figure 8-71 Exudative Open-Funnel Traction Retinal Detachment secondary to Preretinal Membrane in Endophthalmitis, Exudative V-Shaped Posterior Vitreous Detachment with Exudative Vitreoschisis

Horizontal Axial View

This eye has chronic endophthalmitis, with cellular debris permeating all compartments of the eye. Here, there is a V-shaped exudative posterior vitreous detachment, with the nasal side exhibiting a split-hyaloid picture (upper half of the scan) (see Chapter 7). The thickened temporal half, on the other hand, is attached to the preretinal membrane (lower half of the scan). Note that the thick preretinal membrane on the surface of the optic nerve and peripapillary retina has detached the retina on both sides (open-funnel exudative traction retinal detachment). On dynamic examination, the walls of the vitreoschisis undulate, but the thickened half of the hyaloid and the retina remain fixed.

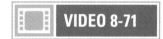

VIDEO 8-71

RETINOSCHISIS

Retinoschisis is a condition where the superficial (inner) layer of the retina splits from its deeper (outer) layer. On ultrasound, however, the thickness of the inner retinal layer does not differ much from that of a full-thickness retina. Retinoschisis is typically dome-shaped, with its base inserted sharply on the ocular wall. It is usually bilateral and often observed at the inferotemporal periphery. Note that cases of retinoschisis resemble dome-shaped, focal RDs echographically. For this reason, information from clinical history and indirect ophthalmoscopy should always be obtained prior to making an ultrasound diagnosis.

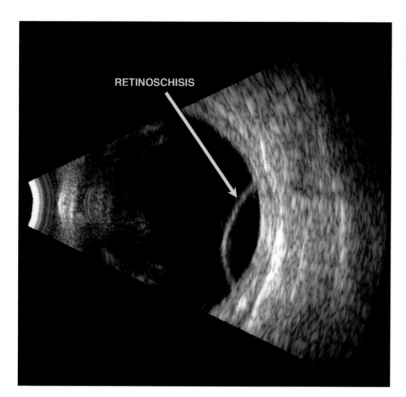

RETINOSCHISIS

Figure 8-72 Retinoschisis

Peripheral Transverse View

On routine fundus examination, this eye was found to have a dome-shaped elevation at the inferotemporal periphery. Here, the retinoschisis jiggles with eye movement.

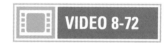

VIDEO 8-72

Figure 8-73   Retinoschisis

Peripheral Transverse View

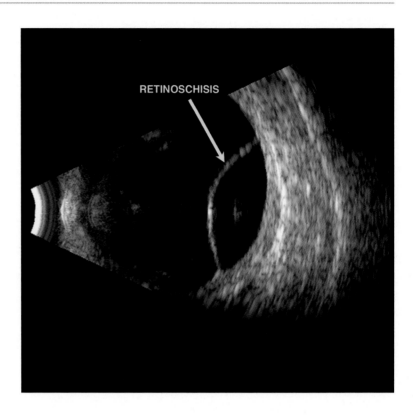

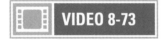

The other eye was also found to have a similar-looking elevation at the inferotemporal periphery. On dynamic examination, the retinoschisis displays an undulating form of aftermovement.

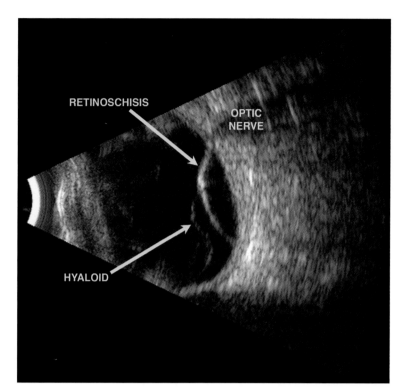

Figure 8-74 Retinoschisis

Horizontal Axial View

Not all cases of retinoschisis are inferotemporal in location. They may occur elsewhere in the fundus. The following scan is obtained from an 86-year-old female with bilateral retinoschisis at the posterior pole. One of her eyes shown here depicts a dome-shaped elevation just temporal to the optic nerve (posterior pole). In this eye, the retinoschisis jiggles as the eye moves.

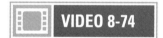

Figure 8-75 Retinoschisis

Peripheral Transverse View

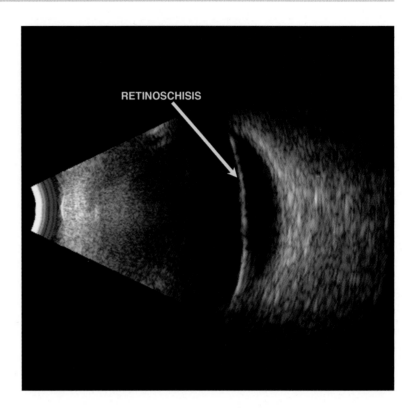

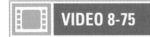

Similarly, not all cases of retinoschisis are dome-shaped. This scan is taken from a 6-year-old boy with bilateral X-linked retinoschisis. One of his eyes displayed here exhibits retinoschisis with a flat, sagging surface. In this eye, the aftermovement is undulating like the hyaloid.

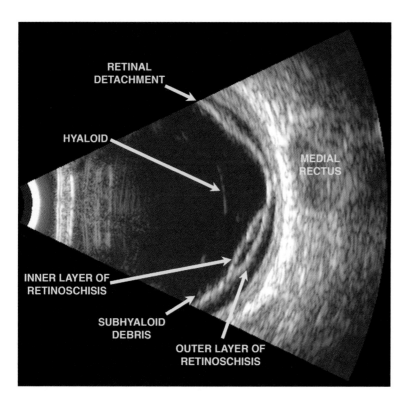

Figure 8-76 Retinoschisis in Retinal Detachment

Transverse View

When the retina is detached, retinoschisis exhibits a split-retina picture. This transverse scan of the nasal retina in a 9-year-old boy demonstrates a low-lying retinal detachment with retinoschisis. On dynamic examination, the retina shakes, whereas the flattened retinoschisis exhibits a more undulating aftermovement similar to the hyaloid. Here, the retina appears cord-like (see Chapter 9). Note that the outer and inner layers of the retinoschisis are almost as thick as the rest of the retinal detachment.

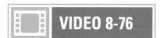

Aftermovement of the Choroid

9

Choroidal detachments (CDs) usually involve the equator and fundus periphery but may extend toward the posterior part of the eye. A CD may be low-lying, where differentiation from retinal detachments (RDs) is mandatory. A CD may also be dome-shaped, where its base is inserted sharply on the scleral wall.

When the choroid detaches from the ocular wall, it actually separates from the sclera along with the retinal layer. For this reason, it appears 2–4 times thicker than RDs, and consequently looks cord-like on ultrasound. It should be noted that in this atlas, the term choroidal detachment loosely refers to detachment of the retinochoroidal complex, as is the case in standard textbooks. However, the term retinochoroidal detachment shall be used in case there is a need to distinguish choroidal detachments that involve the retinochoroidal complex from those that involve the choroid alone.

Low-lying CDs may or may not exhibit a jiggly type of aftermovement. On the other hand, a majority of dome-shaped CDs do not exhibit aftermovement, although some of them may jiggle and a few may shake on dynamic examination.

In this section, we shall look at low-lying and dome-shaped CDs.

> ### TIP
>
> When detached, the choroid is typically cord-like on ultrasound.
>
> **Low-lying CD:** jiggly or no aftermovement
> **Most dome-shaped CDs:** no aftermovement
> **Some dome-shaped CDs:** jiggly, shaky

LOW-LYING CHOROIDAL DETACHMENTS

Low-lying CDs are usually found at the equator and fundus periphery, and they are best viewed on transverse or longitudinal scans. On dynamic examination, they may or may not show a jiggly type of aftermovement. As with low-lying hyaloid and retinal detachments, echographic noise (suprachoroidal artifact) may be observed beneath low-lying CDs, which may masquerade as hemorrhagic, inflammatory, or tumor cells. Suprachoroidal artifacts look like minute echobright streaks, while cellular particles appear more speckled.

Figure 9-1 Low-Lying Serous Choroidal Detachment, Vitreous Debris, and Serous Partial Posterior Vitreous Detachment

Peripheral Transverse View

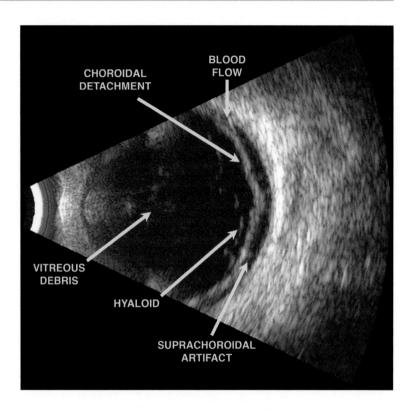

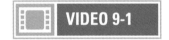

This is a case of low-lying serous choroidal detachment associated with vitreous debris and serous partial posterior vitreous detachment. In this eye, the detached choroid exhibits a cord-like thickness. Here, the choroid jiggles, while the vitreous and hyaloid slowly undulate. Observe the flow of choroidal blood at the upper end of the detachment (see Chapter 5), as well as the presence of a suprachoroidal artifact.

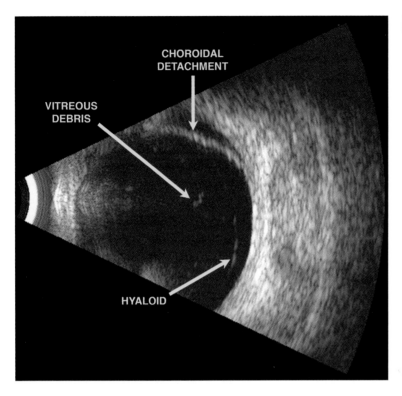

Figure 9-2 Low-Lying Serous Choroidal Detachment, Vitreous Debris, and Serous Partial Posterior Vitreous Detachment

Peripheral Longitudinal View

This is a longitudinal view of the same eye, showing how far anterior or peripheral the detachment is located. Here, the choroid likewise jiggles, whereas the hyaloid undulates.

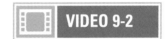

VIDEO 9-2

Figure 9-3 Low-Lying Serous Choroidal Detachment, Vitreous Debris, and Serous Partial Posterior Vitreous Detachment

Peripheral Transverse View

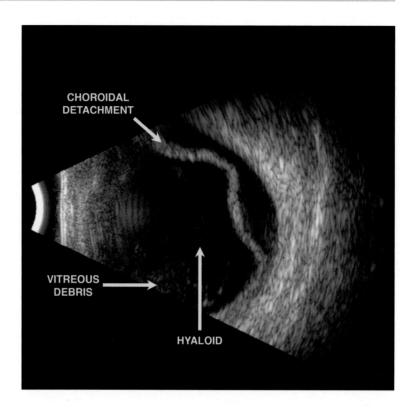

CHOROIDAL DETACHMENT

VITREOUS DEBRIS

HYALOID

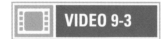 **VIDEO 9-3**

This is another case of low-lying serous choroidal detachment associated with vitreous debris and serous partial posterior vitreous detachment. The periphery of this eye shows a wavy, serous detachment of the choroid. With eye movement, the cord-like choroid jiggles while the hyaloid undulates.

Low-lying CDs may also be associated with RD.

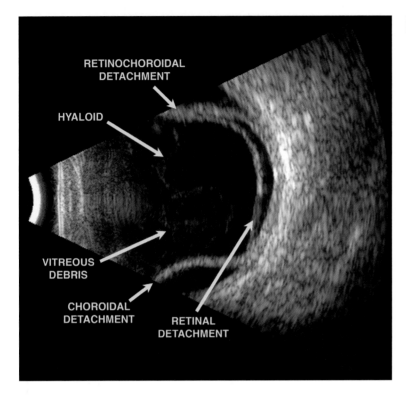

Figure 9-4 Low-Lying Serous Choroidal Detachment, Low-Lying Serous Retinal Detachment, Vitreous Debris, and Serous Partial Posterior Vitreous Detachment

Peripheral Transverse View

This eye presents with low-lying serous choroidal detachment, vitreous debris, and serous partial posterior vitreous detachment, associated with low-lying serous retinal detachment. In this case, the choroidal detachment looks typically cord-like, as opposed to the string-like appearance of the retina. With eye movement, the choroid jiggles, the retina shakes, and the hyaloid undulates.

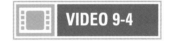
VIDEO 9-4

Figure 9-5 Low-Lying Serous Choroidal Detachment, Focal Serous Retinal Detachment, Vitreous Debris, and Serous Partial Posterior Vitreous Detachment
Peripheral Transverse View

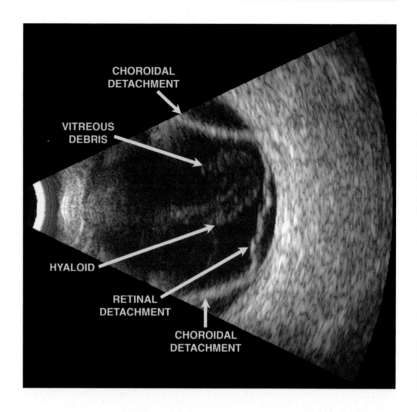

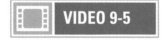

This is another eye with low-lying serous choroidal detachment, vitreous debris, and serous partial posterior vitreous detachment, associated with a focal serous retinal detachment. Here, the detached choroid is typically cord-like, while the wavy retina is string-like. On dynamic examination, the choroid jiggles, the retina gradually shifts, and the hyaloid undulates.

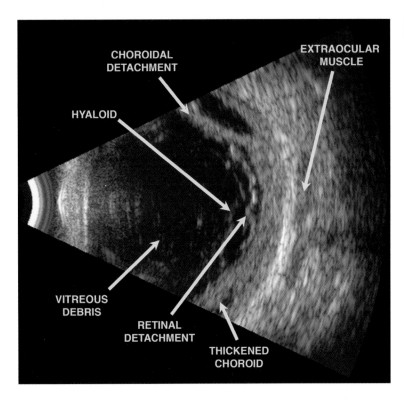

CHOROIDAL DETACHMENT

EXTRAOCULAR MUSCLE

HYALOID

VITREOUS DEBRIS

RETINAL DETACHMENT

THICKENED CHOROID

Figure 9-6 Low-Lying Serous Choroidal Detachment, Low-Lying Serous Retinal Detachment, Vitreous Debris, and Serous Partial Posterior Vitreous Detachment
Peripheral Transverse View

This case depicts low-lying serous choroidal detachment, vitreous debris, and serous partial posterior vitreous detachment, associated with a low-lying and pleated serous retinal detachment. In this example, the retina jiggles with the choroid, whereas the hyaloid undulates. Again, the choroidal detachment appears cord-like and the retina string-like. Note the thickened choroid lining the ocular wall.

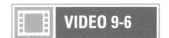

VIDEO 9-6

Figure 9-7 Low-Lying Serous Choroidal Detachment, Low-Lying Serous Retinal Detachment, Vitreous Cells, and Serous Partial Posterior Vitreous Detachment
Peripheral Longitudinal View

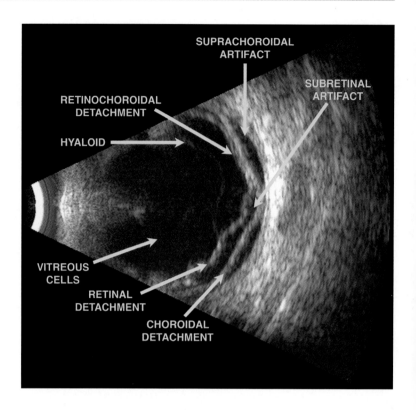

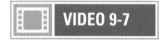

This eye exhibits low-lying serous choroidal detachment, vitreous cells, serous partial posterior vitreous detachment, and low-lying serous retinal detachment. This time, both the retina and the choroid look cord-like, with the former wavy compared to the latter. In this eye, the hyaloid and the retina jiggle, but the choroid remains fixed. Note the subretinal and suprachoroidal artifacts in this scan.

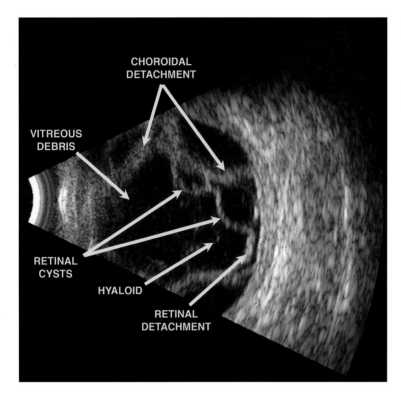

Figure 9-8 Low-Lying Serous Choroidal Detachment, Focal Cystic Serous Retinal Detachment, Vitreous Debris, and Serous Partial Posterior Vitreous Detachment

Peripheral Transverse View

This case presents with low-lying serous choroidal detachment, vitreous debris, and serous partial posterior vitreous detachment. Interestingly, this eye also shows focal, cystic serous retinal detachment as a result of chronic cystic degeneration. In this eye, the retina looks string-like, compared to the cord-like thickness of the choroid. On dynamic examination, the choroid and retina jiggle as the vitreous undulates.

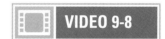

Figure 9-9 Low-Lying Serous Choroidal Detachment, Low-Lying Serous Retinal Detachment, and Vitreous Debris

Peripheral Transverse View

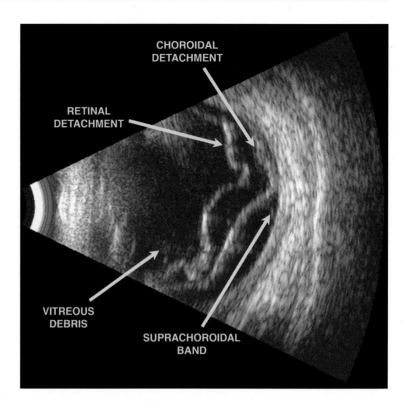

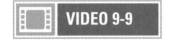
VIDEO 9-9

This eye has low-lying serous choroidal detachment, vitreous debris, and low-lying serous retinal detachment. It demonstrates choroidal detachment and retinal detachment that are momentarily apart from each other. Observe how equally cord-like the retina and choroid are in this example, although the retina appears more folded than the choroid. Here, the choroid jiggles more than the retina. Note that a suprachoroidal band comes into view as the eye moves.

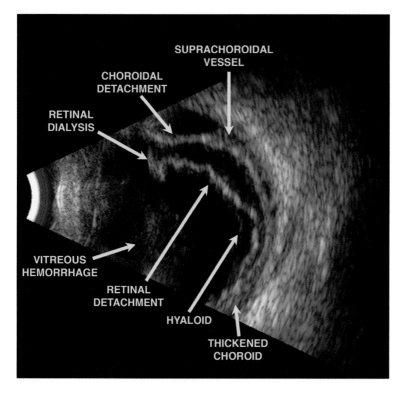

Following traumatic globe rupture, this case exhibited vitreous hemorrhage, low-lying serous choroidal detachment, and retinal detachment. Like the previous example, the choroid and retina in this eye are likewise apart from each other. Note that both choroid and retina are similarly cord-like in appearance. On dynamic examination, the choroid jiggles, whereas the retina undulates with the vitreous and hyaloid. Here, the retina is disinserted from its anterior peripheral attachment, termed retinal dialysis. Observe the flow of blood within the suprachoroidal vessel, as well as the associated choroidal thickening resulting from trauma.

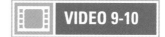

VIDEO 9-10

DOME-SHAPED CHOROIDAL DETACHMENTS

Classically, dome-shaped CDs have taut elevation of the choroid. They typically present without any observable aftermovement.

Figure 9-11 Serous Choroidal Detachment

Horizontal Para-Axial View

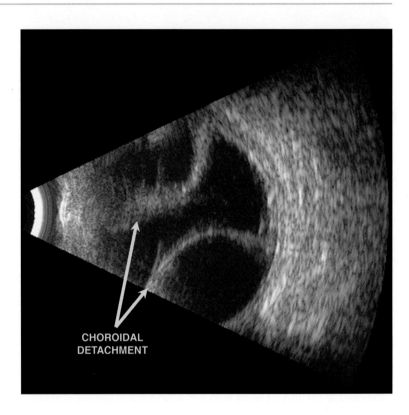

CHOROIDAL
DETACHMENT

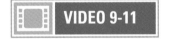 **VIDEO 9-11**

This example demonstrates a bullous type of serous choroidal detachment involving both sides of the equator. Note how distinct and echobright the choroid appears to be, with serous fluid elevating it. Here, the choroid stays rigid during eye movement.

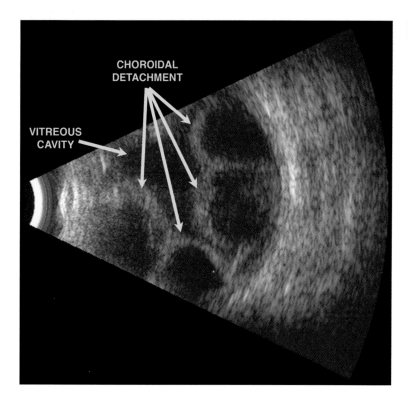

Figure 9-12 Serous Choroidal Detachment
Peripheral Transverse View

This peripheral scan obtained from another eye depicts dome-shaped, serous choroidal detachments that are next to each other. On dynamic examination, choroidal aftermovement is likewise absent.

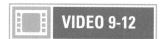

Figure 9-13 Serous Choroidal Detachment

Horizontal Axial View

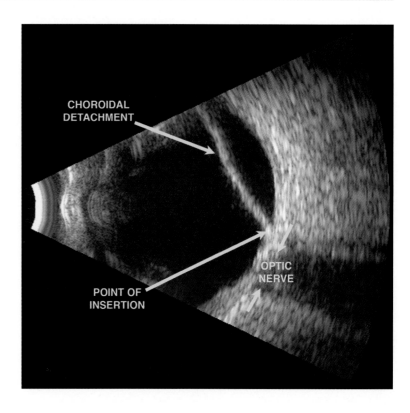

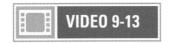 **VIDEO 9-13**

This eye presents with a one-sided and less elevated, serous choroidal detachment. As the eye moves, the choroid displays a jiggly form of aftermovement. Despite its cord-like thickness, this detachment may still be mistaken for the retina, making it necessary to scrutinize the detachment's point of posterior insertion. Retinal detachments insert along the margins of the optic nerve (opposing arrows), whereas choroidal detachments insert just outside its confines.

In hemorrhagic CDs, the choroid appears less defined than its serous counterpart, and somehow blends with blood within the suprachoroidal compartment. Consequently, the elevation tends to look solid like a choroidal mass, especially when there is minimal movement of suprachoroidal blood on dynamic examination.

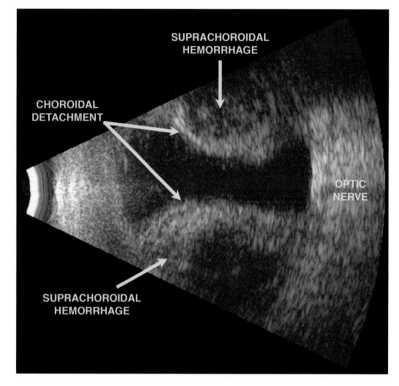

Figure 9-14 Hemorrhagic Choroidal Detachment

Horizontal Para-axial View

This case demonstrates a bullous type of hemorrhagic choroidal detachment involving both sides of the equator. Note that the choroid no longer appears cord-like on account of the suprachoroidal hemorrhage. In this example, no choroidal aftermovement is observed.

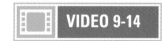

Kissing Choroidal Detachments are an extreme form of dome-shaped CDs. Also termed "kissing choroidals," the choroid from opposite sides of the equator is so elevated that its surfaces become apposed near the central axis of the eye. Posteriorly, these surfaces part just before the surface of the optic nerve, curving outward and inserting on the sclera away from the optic nerve margins. Kissing choroidals should be differentiated from RDs where both sides of the retina insert along the optic nerve margins (see Chapter 8).

Figure 9-15 Hemorrhagic Kissing Choroidal Detachment

Horizontal Axial View

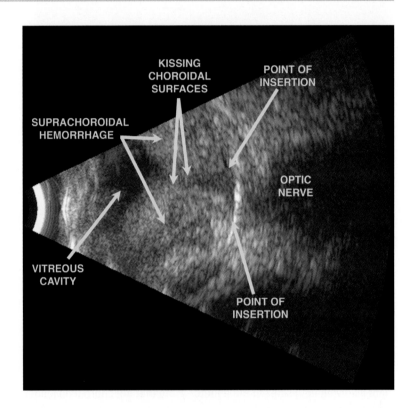

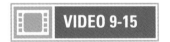

This is a hemorrhagic type of kissing choroidal detachment, where both sides of the choroid separate just before the surface of the optic nerve. Note how the choroid curves outward toward its posterior insertion. During eye movement, blood swirls in the suprachoroidal compartment, but choroidal aftermovement is absent.

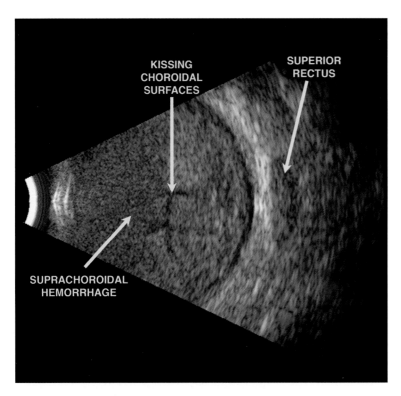

Figure 9-16 Hemorrhagic Kissing Choroidal Detachment
Peripheral Transverse View

This is a transverse scan of another hemorrhagic kissing choroidal detachment, obtained near the insertion of the superior rectus muscle. In this eye, only a fissure-like outline of the apposed choroidal surfaces is seen, surrounded by dense suprachoroidal hemorrhage. On dynamic examination, blood shifts slightly in all compartments, but there is no appreciable choroidal aftermovement.

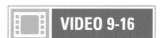

TIP

In kissing choroidal detachments, the "kissing" surfaces part just before the surface of the optic nerve, curve outward, and are inserted on the sclera away from the optic nerve margins.

One should always check the status of the retina in CDs.

Figure 9-17 Serous Choroidal Detachment and Serous Retinal Detachment

Peripheral Transverse View

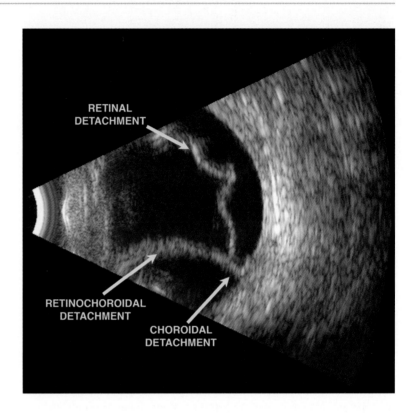

RETINAL
DETACHMENT

RETINOCHOROIDAL
DETACHMENT

CHOROIDAL
DETACHMENT

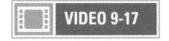 **VIDEO 9-17**

This transverse scan depicts a serous form of choroidal detachment, associated with serous retinal detachment. Here, the retina appears folded. Notice how equally thick the retina and the choroid are, and how much thicker and grainier the retinochoroidal detachment is. With eye movement, the retina reveals a shifting type of aftermovement, whereas the choroid remains rigid.

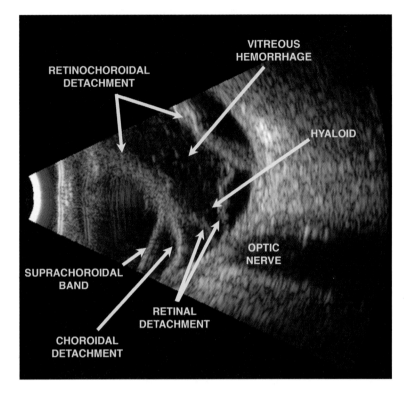

Figure 9-18 Serous Choroidal Detachment, Serous Open-Funnel Retinal Detachment, Vitreous Hemorrhage, and Serous Partial Posterior Vitreous Detachment

Horizontal Axial View

This eye with serous choroidal detachment presents with a serous type of open-funnel retinal detachment. Here, the wavy retina inserts along the margins of the optic nerve, while the choroid curves outward toward its point of attachment. Vitreous hemorrhage, serous partial posterior vitreous detachment, and a suprachoroidal band are likewise seen in this eye. On dynamic examination, the vitreous, hyaloid, and retina shake a bit, but the choroid shows no aftermovement.

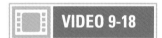

Figure 9-19 Serous Choroidal Detachment, Serous Open-Funnel Retinal Detachment, Vitreous Hemorrhage, and Serous Partial Posterior Vitreous Detachment

Horizontal Axial View

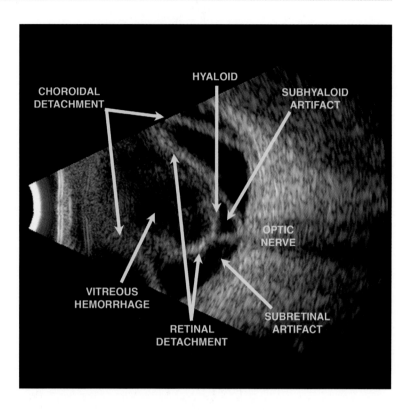

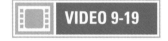

This case of serous choroidal detachment is likewise associated with vitreous hemorrhage, serous partial posterior vitreous detachment, and serous open-funnel retinal detachment. Observe the cord-like thickness of the choroid, retina, and hyaloid. Upon eye movement, the choroid slowly shakes while the vitreous swirls around. However, the hyaloid and the retina remain still. Additionally, note the fleeting presence of subhyaloid and subretinal artifacts in this eye.

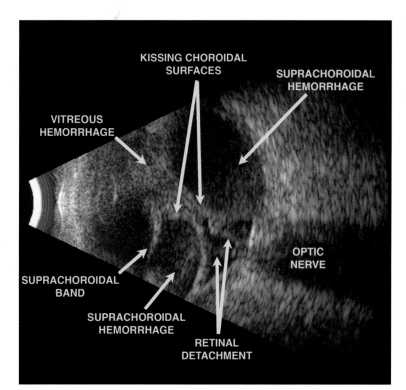

Figure 9-20 Hemorrhagic Kissing Choroidal Detachment and Serous Open-Funnel Retinal Detachment

Horizontal Axial View

This eye has hemorrhagic kissing choroidal detachment. It shows a serous type of open-funnel retinal detachment, depicted by the short V-shaped configuration jutting on the surface of the optic nerve. Vitreous hemorrhage and a suprachoroidal band are also present. With eye movement, both the choroid and retina show no aftermovement. Only the motion of blood can be seen, swirling within the suprachoroidal space.

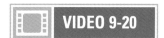

VIDEO 9-20

Figure 9-21 Hemorrhagic Choroidal Detachment and Hemorrhagic Open-Funnel Retinal Detachment due to Giant Retinal Tear

Horizontal Axial View

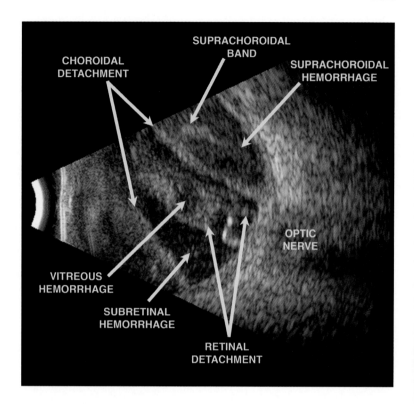

 VIDEO 9-21

This is a post-traumatic case of hemorrhagic choroidal detachment with open-funnel hemorrhagic retinal detachment. Here, the retinal involvement is more obvious than in the previous example, with the retina and choroid looking grainy and cord-like. In this eye, the retina exhibits the zigzag, tortuous profile of retinal detachments secondary to giant retinal tears (see Chapter 8). In addition, vitreous and subretinal hemorrhages, as well as a suprachoroidal band are seen here. On dynamic examination, only the motion of blood in the vitreous and subretinal compartments is discernible, whereas both the retina and choroid stay fixed.

TIP

One should always check the status of the retina in all cases of choroidal detachment.

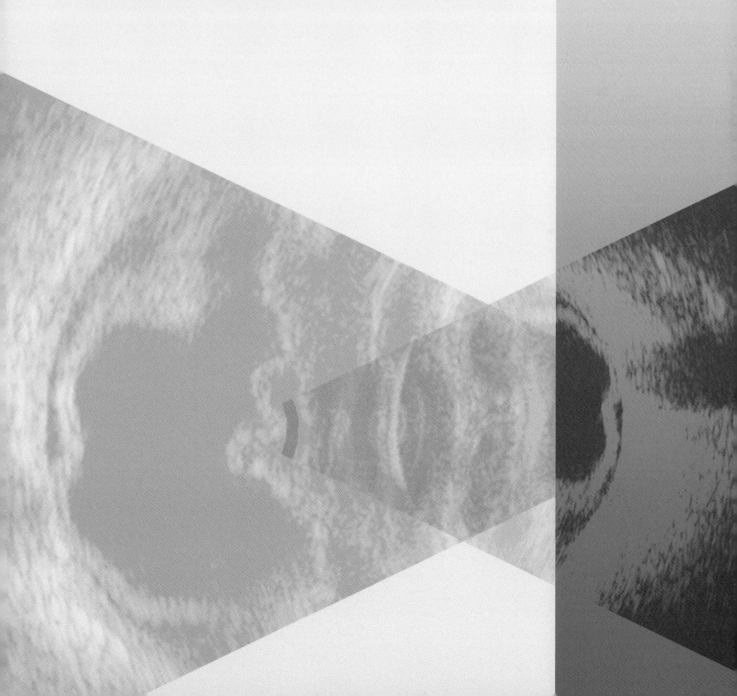

SECTION III

Case Presentations

Complex Dynamic Ultrasound Presentations—Cases

10

COMPLEX DYNAMIC ULTRASOUND PRESENTATIONS

When confronted with a seemingly complicated ultrasound case, one should carefully analyze the scans by performing two basic steps: first, identify the ophthalmic tissues involved, and second, observe how these tissues move about in relation to the other associated findings. If these steps are routinely followed, one should be able to arrive at the right diagnosis in a systematic and logical manner. In this section, six cases are presented to the reader to gauge what has been learned from the previous chapters.

CASE 1

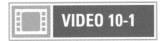

This is a dynamic horizontal axial scan of a 49-year-old male, referred to this institution for evaluation of the eye. A month prior to consultation, he underwent surgery of a ruptured globe immediately following a shotgun injury to the face. Vision was hand motion at the time of ultrasound examination.

Watch Video 10-1, and then record your observations and/or impressions before proceeding.

Figure 10-1

Horizontal Axial View

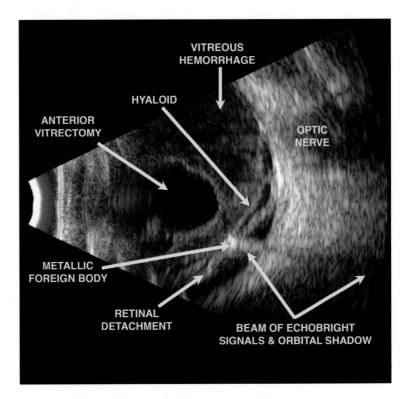

The temporal detachment appears cord-like (lower half of the scan). In front of it is a string-like detachment, with residual attachment to the optic nerve margins and the nasal retina (upper half of the scan). These two detachments are stuck together by a hyperechoic spot midway along the temporal detachment. This spot casts a flared beam of echobright signals and orbital shadow posteriorly, typical of metallic intraocular foreign bodies (see Fig. 7-18). On dynamic examination, the cord-like detachment shakes and is noted to insert at the lower margin of the optic nerve. These observations point to a retinal involvement. The string-like detachment, on the other hand, undulates with the vitreous, which is a hyaloid trait. Note the scooped appearance of the anterior vitreous, which was subsequently confirmed to be a consequence of previous anterior vitrectomy.

DIAGNOSIS

Case 1: Low-lying Temporal Retinal Detachment with Incarcerated Hyaloid secondary to Metallic Intraocular Foreign Body, Vitreous Hemorrhage, and Serous Partial Posterior Vitreous Detachment status post Anterior Vitrectomy and Ruptured Globe Repair.

CASE 2

This is a dynamic horizontal axial scan of an 83-year-old female with chronic poor vision of hand motion. She was referred for evaluation of the posterior ocular segment.

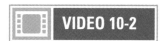

Watch Video 10-2, and then record your observations and/or impressions before proceeding.

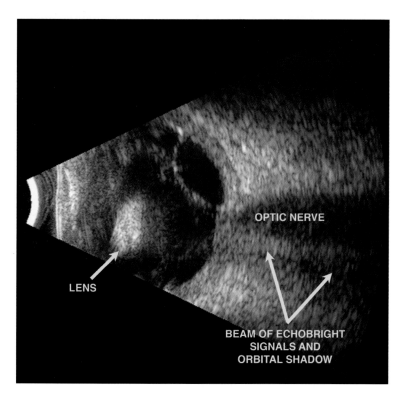

Figure 10-2A

Horizontal Axial View

The hyperechoic, coin-like mass tumbling to and fro in the posterior vitreous is a dislocated cataractous lens, shown in an en-face orientation. It casts a flared beam of echobright signals and orbital shadow towards the back (see Chapter 3). Notice how this beam alternately blocks the view of the optic nerve and the macula (lower half of the scan) as the lens gravitates toward these areas.

Next, examine the dome-shaped elevation just nasal to the surface of the optic nerve (upper half of the scan) (see Video 10-2).

Horizontal Axial View

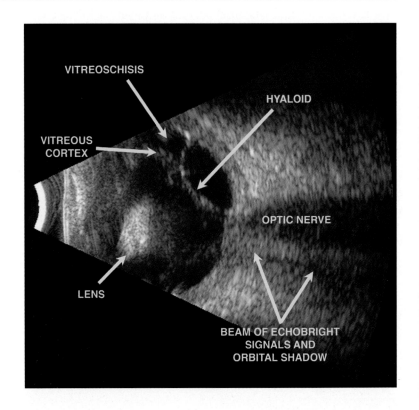

This dome-shaped elevation looks like a focal retinal detachment on account of its string-like appearance. As the eye moves, however, it displays an undulating form of aftermovement, which is characteristically hyaloid. Furthermore, a split-hyaloid image is observed next to it (top side of the scan) (see Chapter 7).

Initially, this case is diagnosed to be Posterior Lens Dislocation and Serous Partial Posterior Vitreous Detachment with Vitreoschisis.

Remember, though, that the macula should always be checked whenever ultrasonography is performed, especially when its view is shadowed or obstructed by a dislocated lens. Hence, during the course of dynamic examination, the patient's head was elevated to shift the lens away from the posterior pole by gravity. Horizontal axial scanning was then repeated.

Watch Video 10-3.

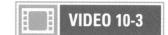

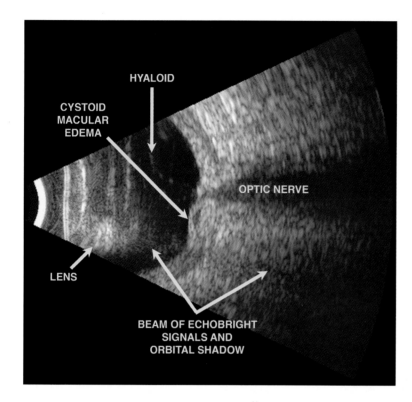

Figure 10-3

Horizontal Axial View

As the eye moves from side to side, the beam cast by the cataractous lens alternately blocks and clears the view of the posterior pole. This time, a fixed elevated macula is uncovered, which is, in fact, cystoid macular edema.

DIAGNOSIS

Case 2: Posterior Lens Dislocation, Serous Partial Posterior Vitreous Detachment with Vitreoschisis, and Cystoid Macular Edema.

CASE 3

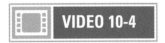

This is a dynamic horizontal axial scan of a 56-year-old male, referred for retinal evaluation following repair of a ruptured globe in another institution. He presented with an 8-ball hyphema, and the eye had no light perception.

Watch Video 10-4, and then record your observations and/or impressions before proceeding.

Figure 10-4A

Horizontal Axial View

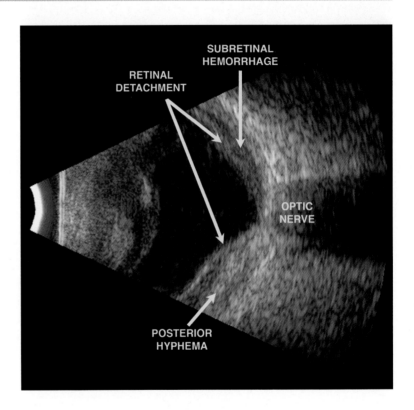

At first glance, this eye appears to be filled with vitreous hemorrhage, with either a hemorrhagic choroidal effusion or a low-lying hemorrhagic open-funnel detachment. Upon eye movement, the cord-like detachment displays a shifting type of aftermovement. This is a retinal, and not a choroidal, tissue attribute (see Chapter 8). Note the formation of a posterior hyphema, and observe the motion of subretinal cells.

Next, observe the anterior part of the eye (see Video 10-4).

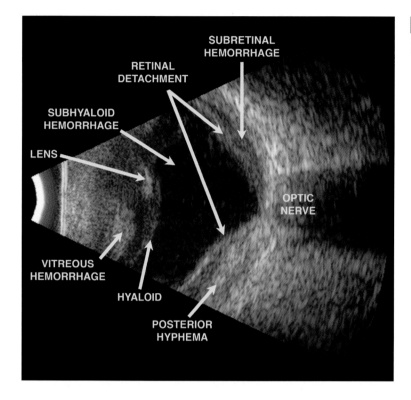

Figure 10-4B

Horizontal Axial View

Just behind the lens is the anteriorly retracted hyaloid, appearing grainy from vitreous hemorrhage and showing some shakiness during eye movement (see Chapter 7). Hence, blood dispersed in front of the retinal detachment is really subhyaloid hemorrhage and not vitreous hemorrhage as previously thought.

DIAGNOSIS

Initial Diagnosis for Case 3: Hemorrhagic Complete Posterior Vitreous Detachment with Vitreous Hemorrhage, Hemorrhagic Retinal Detachment status post Ruptured Globe Repair.

TIP

Whenever vitreous, subhyaloid, or subretinal hemorrhage is present in the eye, one should always attempt to look for its source.

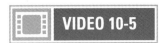 **VIDEO 10-5**

This time, watch Video 10-5, which is a transverse view of the inferior periphery.

Figure 10-5

Inferior Peripheral Transverse View

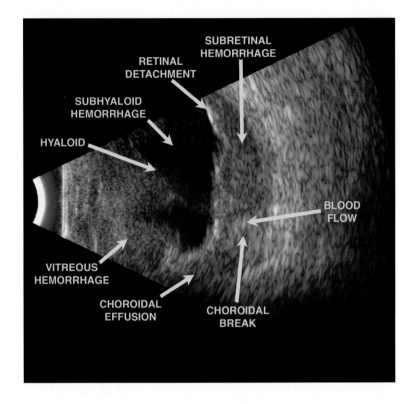

Part of both hyaloid and retinal detachments is shown in this scan. Likewise, a hemorrhagic type of choroidal effusion is observed next to the retinal detachment (lower half of the scan). More significantly, this view reveals active bleeding at the junction of the retinal detachment and choroidal effusion, approximately where the choroidal break appears to have occurred (see Chapter 5).

DIAGNOSIS

Final Diagnosis for Case 3: Hemorrhagic Complete Posterior Vitreous Detachment with Vitreous Hemorrhage, Hemorrhagic Retinal Detachment and Hemorrhagic Choroidal Effusion secondary to Active Choroidal Bleeding status post Ruptured Globe Repair.

CASE 4

This is a dynamic horizontal axial scan of a 56-year-old male with corneal ulcer. He was referred for ultrasound examination to rule out endophthalmitis.

Watch Video 10-6, and then record your observations and/or impressions before proceeding.

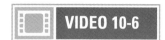

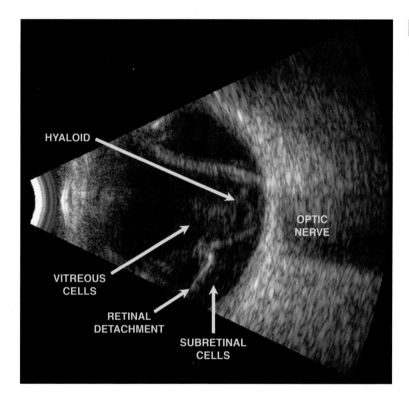

Figure 10-6A

Horizontal Axial View

In this eye, the vitreous is filled with cellular debris, with the hyaloid partially detached and undulating. Note that a chunk of the vitreous and hyaloid still adheres to the surface of the optic nerve. More importantly, there is a wide, V-shaped configuration that seems to be an open-funnel retinal detachment. On closer inspection, the temporal side appears more folded, string-like, and somewhat grainy from the effect of cells underneath the detachment (lower half of the scan). Additionally, it is inserted along the lower margin of the optic nerve and displays a shaky aftermovement. These findings are consistent with a retinal tissue involvement.

Next, examine the nasal side (upper half of the scan) (see Video 10-6).

Figure 10-6B

Horizontal Axial View

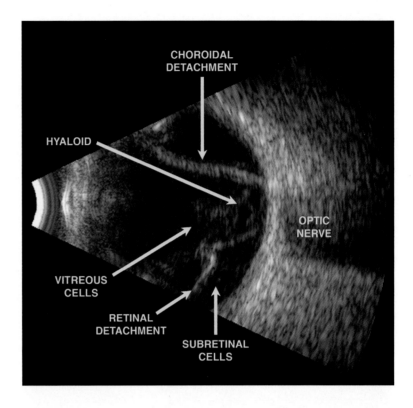

The nasal detachment appears much thicker and cord-like compared to the temporal side, and it is actually inserted on the ocular wall just outside the upper margin of the optic nerve. These observations point to a choroidal, and not a retinal, tissue involvement. Here, the choroid demonstrates a shaky aftermovement, with clear, serous fluid filling the suprachoroidal space.

DIAGNOSIS

Case 4: Serous Partial Posterior Vitreous Detachment, Temporal Exudative Retinal Detachment, and Nasal Serous Choroidal Detachment in Endophthalmitis.

CASE 5

This is a dynamic horizontal axial scan of a 53-year-old diabetic female with dense vitreous hemorrhage. She was referred for assessment of the retina.

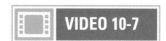

Watch Video 10-7, and then record your observations and/or impressions before proceeding.

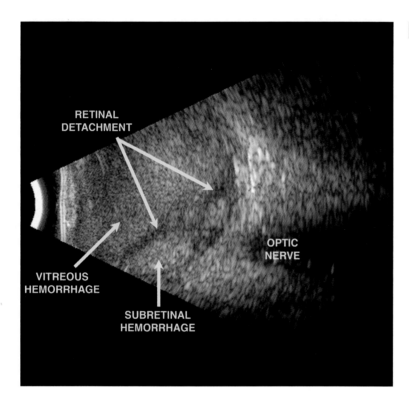

Figure 10-7A

Horizontal Axial View

In this eye, the profusion of hemorrhage in the vitreous cavity basically masks the fundus findings. Nevertheless, the silhouette of a relatively echolucent low-lying, open-funnel retinal detachment could be seen in front of the optic nerve (see Chapter 8). On dynamic examination, vitreous blood swirls in a wave-like fashion, subretinal hemorrhage shifts from side to side, but the echolucent retina shows no aftermovement.

Next, examine the nasal equator (top side of the scan) (see Video 10-7).

Figure 10-7B

Horizontal Axial View

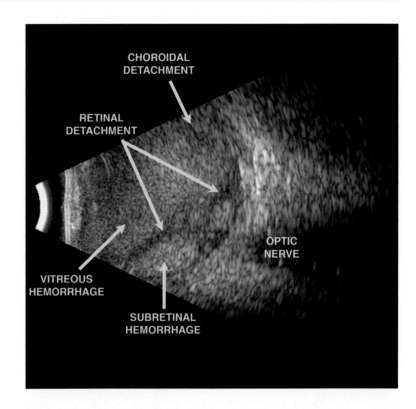

Here, a mound of hemorrhagic choroidal detachment is barely apparent. However, no choroidal aftermovement is discernible. As the eye moves back and forth, note the counterflow of suprachoroidal blood vis-à-vis the direction of flow of the vitreous hemorrhage.

DIAGNOSIS

Case 5: Vitreous Hemorrhage, Hemorrhagic Open-Funnel Retinal Detachment, and Nasal Hemorrhagic Choroidal Detachment.

CASE 6

This is a dynamic horizontal axial scan of a 40-year-old male with no view of the fundus, referred for ultrasound imaging of the posterior segment.

Watch Video 10-8, and then record your observations and/or impressions before proceeding.

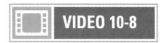

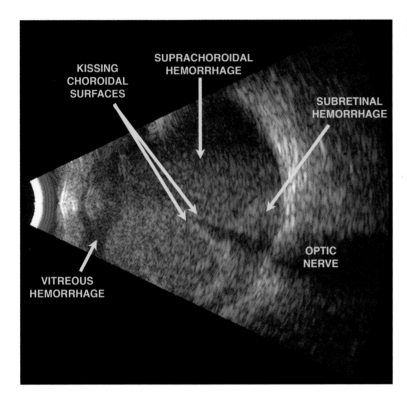

Figure 10-8A

Horizontal Axial View

This scan is reminiscent of a kissing type of hemorrhagic choroidal detachment (see Chapter 9). On dynamic examination, blood swirls within the nasal side of the eye (upper half of the scan), as well as the anterior vitreous compartment.

Next, look at the area in front of the optic nerve (see Video 10-8).

(see Video 10-8)

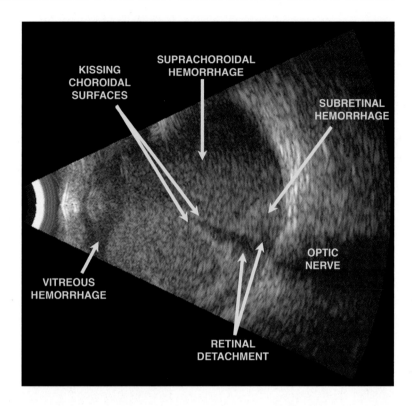

Figure 10-8B

Horizontal Axial View

As you look closely in front of the optic nerve, the kissing choroidal surfaces part, curve sideways, and are inserted on the wall away from the optic nerve. At the point of choroidal separation, however, another pair of detachments can be seen continuing posteriorly towards the optic nerve. This is actually the base of a very narrow open-funnel retinal detachment, appearing echolucent from the effect of dense hemorrhage beneath the detachment (see Chapter 8). Here, the retina shakes a bit during eye movement.

Now, shift your attention to the lower half of the scan (see Video 10-8).

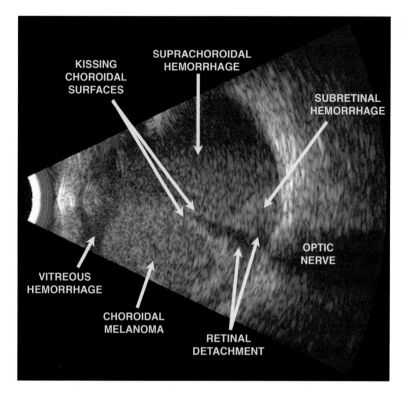

Figure 10-8C

Horizontal Axial View

On dynamic examination, the temporal side of the eye (lower half of the scan) looks solid compared to the other half. More importantly, one can observe the shimmering motion going on within the mass (see Chapter 5). This is a classic sign of choroidal melanoma.

DIAGNOSIS

Case 6: Vitreous Hemorrhage, Hemorrhagic Retinal Detachment, and Hemorrhagic Kissing Choroidal Detachment secondary to Choroidal Melanoma.

TIP

In hemorrhagic kissing choroidal detachments, one should always check for the presence of a choroidal mass.

Based on the preceding examples, ultrasound scans appear complex when several ophthalmic findings present at the same time, along with a simultaneous display of tissue movements. To make matters worse, ophthalmic tissues no longer look typical, and their movements have become modified by the coexisting changes. In short, the barrage of visual information overloads the viewer. Consequently, one is drawn to whatever feature dominates the ultrasound picture, with a tendency to overlook associated findings that are subtle and inconspicuous, yet critical to the management of a case.

Case 1 could have been misdiagnosed as CD with incarcerated retina instead of RD with incarcerated hyaloid secondary to a metallic intraocular foreign body, had the resident relied solely on the appearance of the tissues instead of observing its respective movements on dynamic B-scan. Case 2 could have been misconstrued to be associated with a focal RD, had the examiner taken the detachment to be of a retinal and not hyaloid nature. Additionally, the status of the macula could not have been verified had there been a lack of awareness about the intense shadowing effect of dislocated cataractous lenses on structures located behind them. Case 3 could have been thought to be stable following repair of the ruptured globe, had the technician not vigorously looked for the source of the vitreous, subhyaloid, and subretinal hemorrhages. Case 4 could have been misinterpreted solely as an open-funnel RD, had the doctor not closely observed the differences in thickness, insertion, and tissue behavior between the nasal and temporal detachments. Case 5 could have been misjudged to be plain VH with posterior hyphema, had the ultrasonographer not scrutinized the area in front of the optic nerve and the equator, where RD and CD, respectively, were barely noticeable. Case 6 could have been misdiagnosed to be another case of hemorrhagic kissing CD, had the practitioner not reviewed the dynamic scans very carefully. For this final case, uncovering a huge malignant tumor thriving in an eye that presents as a kissing type of hemorrhagic CD totally changes its prognosis and management.

In all of these examples, we looked at the overall picture initially. Next, we focused at each finding, proceeding from the most to the least dominant change that each scan presented. We then observed the appearance of each finding, and watched the movements closely. Lastly, we correlated each of our observations to the overall picture.

Ultimately, the key to becoming astute at ultrasound analysis is to be thorough in examining each case. One should sift through the complexity by studying each finding meticulously and by observing each movement repeatedly, until a clear general picture of the ophthalmic pathology emerges. Certainly, having a firm knowledge of all possible variations in tissue behavior could help refine one's ability to interpret these scans, so that proper and timely management can be delivered without delay.

Limitations of Dynamic Ophthalmic Ultrasonography

11

By and large, each case included in the atlas, from the most basic to the most complex presentation, demonstrated variations in the appearance of ophthalmic tissues. A considerable number showed similar or identical ultrasound images, but most of them could be differentiated by closely observing the behavior of tissues on dynamic B-scan examinations. Still, a few remained starkly alike and indistinguishable from each other despite the study of motion, such as vitreous hemorrhage and endophthalmitis, retinoschisis and dome-shaped focal retinal detachment, low-lying peripheral hyaloid detachment and low-lying peripheral retinal detachment, as well as V-shaped posterior vitreous detachment and open-funnel retinal detachment. For these few exceptions, the clinical history as well as findings on indirect ophthalmoscopy should help resolve the differential diagnosis. Without these, definite ultrasound diagnosis cannot be made.

Post-traumatic eyes pose the greatest challenge to performing useful, confirmatory dynamic ultrasound scans. In this setting, the eye is congested, the lids are swollen and shut, and the patient is usually in great pain. Additionally, ocular movement is minimal because of guarding, which prevents the examiner from actually observing and detecting which intraocular tissues have been affected and damaged by the traumatic event. There is really nothing much one can do, except to image the eye as best as possible, in the least painful manner, during the initial visit. The procedure should then be performed at a more favorable time when ocular inflammation has subsided, and the patient is more receptive to undergoing a more thorough, dynamic ultrasound examination.

Bibliography

1. Greene, R., & Byrne, S. F. (2002). *Ultrasound of the eye and orbit*. (2nd ed.). Philadelphia: Mosby.
2. Rosen, R. B., Dunne, S., & Garcia, J. P. S. (2003). 3D-Ultrasound tomography. In Ciulla, T., Regillo, C., & Harris, A. (Eds.), *Retina and optic nerve imaging*. Philadelphia: Lippincott Williams & Wilkins.
3. Garcia, J. P. S., Jr., Garcia, P. M. T, & Finger, P. T. (2006). Dynamic ultrasound movements of the eye and orbit. *British Journal of Ophthalmology*, 90, 395–520. Available at http://bjo.bmjjournals.com/cgi/content/full/90/4/DC1/1?eaf. Accessed April 16, 2009.
4. Garcia, J. P. S., Jr., Garcia, P. M. T., & Rosen, R. B. (2005). Wide-field handheld high-frequency ultrasonography using the new OTI HF 35–50 high frequency ultrasound system. *Ophthalmic Surgery Lasers and Imaging*, 36, 139–141.

SUGGESTED READINGS

Greene, R., & Byrne, S. F. (2002). *Ultrasound of the eye and orbit*. (2nd ed.). Philadelphia: Mosby.

Coleman, D. J., Silverman, R. H., Lizzi, F. L., et al. (2005). *Ultrasonography of the eye and orbit*. (2nd ed.). Philadelphia: Lippincott Williams & Wilkins.

DiBernardo, C. W., & Greenberg, E. (2006). *Ophthalmic ultrasound. A diagnostic atlas*. (2nd ed.). New York: Thieme Medical Publishers.

Pavlin, C. J., & Foster, F. S. (1995). *Ultrasound biomicroscopy of the eye*. New York: Springer-Verlag.

Chapter 5 | Vascularity

Chapter 6 | Aftermovement of the Vitreous

Chapter 7 | Aftermovement of the Hyaloid

Chapter 8 | Aftermovement of the Retina

Closed-Funnel Retinal Detachments

Chapter 9 | Aftermovement of the Choroid

Low-Lying Choroidal Detachments

Chapter 10 | Complex Dynamic Ultrasound Presentations—Cases

Chapter 11 | Limitations of Dynamic Ophthalmic Ultrasonography

(no videos)